MALE SEXUAL AWARE- NESS

Increasing Sexual Satisfaction

D0449186

MALE SEXUAL AWARE- NESS

Increasing Sexual Satisfaction

BARRY McCARTHY

Carroll & Graf Publishers, Inc.
New York

Copyright © 1988 by Barry McCarthy

All rights reserved

First Carroll & Graf edition 1988

Second Printing 1989

Carroll & Graf Publishers, Inc
260 Fifth Avenue
New York, NY 10001

Library of Congress Cataloging-in-Publication Data

McCarthy, Barry W., 1943–
 Male sexual awareness.

 1. Men—Sexual behavior. 2. Sex. I. Title.
HQ28.M29 1988   613.9′6′ 088375   87-25598
ISBN 0-88184-348-2 (pbk.)

Manufactured in the United States of America

Table of Contents

To my children
Mark Matthew, Kara Dawn
and Paul Trevor

1
THE MYTH OF THE
MALE PERFORMANCE MACHINE

If you are male and have started reading this, it is probably because you think there might be something about male sexuality that you don't know. If you happen to be in a bookstore or have found this book on a friend's coffee table, and there are people present who may be watching you as you read, chances are that you are feeling self-conscious. After all, men aren't supposed to have to read about sex. They are expected to know all there is to know. Acknowledging that there is still something left to learn is a sign of weakness, an admission that you are not the man you ought to be.

It is a pity that so many men feel this way, because the present era is unparalleled in the amount of information that has come to light on human sexuality. Surveys and laboratory studies have provided definitive answers to questions about human sexual functioning and behavior that for years were matters of conjecture. The herculean investigations of Dr. Alfred Kinsey demonstrated that the sexual activity of most of us was neither excessive nor unusual, but fit comfortably into a wide spectrum of normality. After Kinsey, it became plain that everyone had a sex life, a fact that had often been cast in doubt during the long sexual cover-up of the Victorian age. Another great milestone came with the publications of Dr. William H. Masters and Virginia E. Johnson. Using an array of medical testing instruments as well as video recordings in a laboratory setting, these pioneering sex researchers studied the physiological responses of volunteers engaging in sexual intercourse and a variety of other sexual interactions. From this innovative method

1

of investigation came a wealth of fresh data on the ways in which humans actually respond to sexual stimulation. With the publication of Masters and Johnson's "Human Sexual Inadequacy" in 1970, we gained an understanding not only of sexual response but also of how to deal with sexual dysfunction and promote more pleasurable sexual experiences. Since 1970 there has been a wealth of professional and general books published on virtually all aspects of human sexuality.

"But what does that have to do with me?" you may ask. The answer is that the findings about human sexuality are important to all of us. Although sexuality is a natural, physiological function, our sexual attitudes, behaviors, and emotional reactions are learned. Our sexuality can be a source of great pleasure, a means of intimate communication, an expression of joy in a relationship—or it can be a cause of pain and unhappiness. Whether sex has a positive or negative effect on our lives depends at least in part on whether our sexual attitudes are based on ignorance and misinformation or on facts. Obtaining accurate information about sex is the first step in making a good sexual adjustment.

HOW MUCH DO YOU REALLY KNOW ABOUT MALE SEXUALITY?

Unfortunately, few of us are really well informed about sex. It has been estimated that only about one out of six men in our society has received an adequate sex education. Despite the fact that the subject of sex seems to permeate our society, sexual myths and misconceptions continue to be prevalent. Many generally well informed and sophisticated men unquestionably accept certain beliefs about sexuality that are, in fact, completely untrue. If you wonder about your own sexual knowledge, you might find it instructive to take the following test. Simply read each statement and indicate whether it is true or false.

1. The size of a man's penis is an indication of the strength of his sex drive.
2. The larger the penis, the greater the stimulation for the woman during intercourse.
3. A man's sexuality peaks during adolescence. After the age of twenty, his sexual ability, his interest, and his enjoyment of sex all decline.

4. It is natural for a man to be interested chiefly in intercourse and orgasm. Foreplay and affectionate touching appeal mostly to women.
5. The ability to ejaculate rapidly is a sign of masculinity.
6. If you have experienced the inability to maintain an erection once, it is likely that you will develop a major sex problem.
7. The extent of a man's success in his first intercourse experience is usually an indication of how successful he will be during the rest of his sexual life.
8. On the average, black men have larger penises than white men and also have a stronger sex drive.
9. Masturbation is detrimental to a man's sexual ability.
10. A liking for oral-genital sex is a sign of immaturity.
11. Male and female sexual responses are essentially different from one another.
12. Having homosexual fantasaies or feeling attraction for other men is usually a sign of latent homosexuality.
13. Homosexuality is considered a form of mental illness.
14. The most natural position for sexual intercourse is the male on top.
15. A healthy, well-adjusted man should have no trouble performing sexually in any situation.
16. Since conception takes place in the woman's body, it is her responsibility to prevent an unwanted pregnancy.
17. Erection is always a sign of sexual excitement and indicates a need for intercourse.
18. A good lover is able to give his partner an orgasm each time they have intercourse.
19. Some men are just naturally better lovers than others. While you may be able to learn certain sexual skills, you will never be able to match the performance of someone who has more inborn ability than you do.
20. Simultaneous orgasm is the most fulfilling sexual goal for a couple.
21. The normal frequency of intercourse for a couple in their twenties or early thirties is four times a week. Having intercourse less often indicates that you have a low sex drive.
22. Sexual intercourse should be avoided during menstruation and pregnancy.

23. Men who have suffered a heart attack or a stroke are better off avoiding intercourse.
24. Women respond to sexual stimulation much more slowly than men and must be "worked on" by their partner to get them ready for intercourse.
25. When a man reaches adulthood, he loses interest in fantasy and masturbation and concentrates exclusively on intercourse.

If you answered true for any of the above statements, then there are things you can learn about sexuality, because every one of the twenty-five statements is false. They are all common sex myths, many of which are widely accepted to this day despite overwhelming evidence to the contrary. They have led to incalculable dissatisfaction, frustration, insecurity, and misunderstanding for both men and women.

MALE RESISTANCE TO SEX INFORMATION

But while inaccurate information about sex is detrimental to both men and women, it is men who are more likely to perpetuate and cling to the old sex myths. Because men are expected to be sexual experts, it is difficult for them to admit that they might be wrong or misinformed. Because they cannot admit their ignorance, they will not allow themselves to ask questions and to be receptive to sexual information. And in the absence of accurate information, the old and damaging sex myths are perpetuated ad infintium.

One of the real paradoxes about sexuality is that in our generation the people wisest about it aren't men but women. For women are far more open than we are to information and advice on sexuality. They are far more willing to admit their lack of knowledge and expertise, while we tend to be convinced that what we don't already know isn't worth learning. Women, on the other hand, are more aware that there is room for improvement.

Walk into any bookstore or library and look at the books on sexuality. You will see many volumes for, by, and about women, but few devoted to the subject of male sexuality. The receptivity of women to advice on sexuality is well known. Publishers assume (and not without reason) that men will turn away from such books with a shrug of "Who needs it? I know it already."

The majority of books on male sexuality are actually bought and read by women, not men.

It is not only in bookstores that one sees evidence of the male know-it-all attitude toward sex. I have encountered it many times in my work as a college professor. For seventeen years I have taught a course in human sexual behavior in the psychology department at a large metropolitan university. Not only do roughly four times as many female students enroll in the course, but males tend to ask fewer questions and rarely take part in class discussions. The female students are no more embarrassed to reveal their incomplete knowledge of human sexual behavior than they would be to confess their ignorance of organic chemistry or English literature. As a result, they derive far greater benefit from the course.

PERSONAL RELUCTANCE TO DISCUSS SEXUALITY

This reluctance on the part of most men to learn about sex from books or in classroom situations extends to an uneasiness about exchanging sexual information on a personal basis. Few fathers are able to communicate freely with their sons about human sexuality. Far too often, sex is a taboo subject in the home until the father finally decides that it is time for him to inform his son about the "facts of life," or to give him a package of condoms and tell him to stay out of trouble. This father-son confrontation often takes the form of a brief, awkward lecture that answers only such basic questions as who puts what where, if even that. Since the father himself probably harbors many misconceptions about sex, he is likely to pass these on to his son. Moreover, since the son has been discouraged from thinking of his parents as sexual beings all his life, and because he senses his father's discomfort, he is unwilling to ask questions in order to clarify the points he does not understand. He, like his father, pretends he is knowledgeable.

The reluctance to discuss sex frankly and openly affects other male relationships. It is rare to find young males who are truthful with each other about their first sex experiences. The best available statistics show that about 25 percent of all males are unsuccessful in their first intercourse, generally because they fail to achieve or maintain an erection or because they ejaculate before the penis enters the vagina. One out of four is a substantial proportion, enough to make the experience a common one. And yet, can you imagine the following dialogue taking place?

"Hey, Jimmy, how'd it go with Harriet last night?"

"Not too good, Fred. I came before I could get in."

"Well, don't worry about it, Jim. You'll do better next time."

It is far more likely that Jimmy would claim that he had performed like a prize bull, even if his experience with Harriet had been the fiasco of his young life. He would claim Harriet was so impressed with him sexually that she'd pay him to have sex with her. Or, if Jimmy were so foolish as to admit that he had had an erection or premature ejaculation problem, it is probable that Fred would never let him hear the end of it. We are not kind to each other where sex is concerned. People who harbor anxieties and insecurities rarely are.

LIVING UP TO MALE PERFORMANCE DEMANDS

Thus, most men end up cheating themselves out of a great deal of sexual pleasure. Not only are we expected to be sexually knowledgeable without having received adequate instruction, but we are expected to perform flawlessly at every sexual opportunity. Trying to live up to these impossible demands is likely to cause anxiety and insecurity. For many men, sex is a bluff, a desperate struggle to maintain the image of the infallible "male performance machine." When sex becomes so competitive, so performance oriented, there is little room for pleasure.

The size of our equipment, the number of times we can come—these are the things that concern us, not how much enjoyment we give and receive during the sexual experience. Most destructive of all is the notion that we must never default, never fail to perform. According to the commonly accepted standard, a "real man" is able and willing to have sex anytime, anywhere, with any available female. It rarely occurs to us that the ability to meet such demands is simply not human. Absolute reliability is a standard that should be applied to machines, not people. And yet, this is precisely what we demand of ourselves.

The time has come for us to escape from the rigid and oppressive male image that has for so long prevented us from fully enjoying our sexuality. Women have already begun slough-ing off their socially imposed image, and we can learn a great deal from their example. The object of the feminist movement is not to put down men but to alter the confining and rigid roles that frustrate both men and women. As a result of this effort, there has been an awakening of women's sense of themselves as autonomous beings, in control of and responsible for their own sexuality. It is a shame that many men feel threatened by women who insist on being equal both as people and as sex partners. The most enjoyable sexual experiences result when both the man and woman are able to understand and express their own sexual needs as well as respond to those of their partner.

The object of this book is not to transform the reader into a superlover whose performance will leave his partners panting for more. Understanding a woman's anatomy and pattern of response and knowing the kinds of stimulation that are most effective in producing arousal and orgasm are necessary aspects of being a good lover, but they are not the most important. A good lover is not a technician; he is someone who can enjoy and be involved in the feelings of tenderness, intimacy, and emo-tional expression that occur during sexual interaction. In addi-tion to knowing how to give pleasure, he is able to accept it as well. He sees himself as deserving of pleasure, and he under-stands that lovemaking is not just a skill to be practiced within the confines of the bedroom, but rather is one expression of a general feeling of comfort, affection, and communication be-tween partners. He adopts the view that sex is good, not bad, and that his sexuality is more than his penis, intercourse, and orgasm—it is a positive integral part of his personality. This man wants sexuality to enhance his life and intimate relation-ship, not cause confusion, guilt, and trauma.

WHAT THIS BOOK IS ABOUT

Thus, the purpose of this book is twofold. It is to present the most accurate, reliable information presently available on male sexuality and on topics related to sexual functioning. Second, it is to help men integrate their sexuality with the rest of their lives in a way that will bring them greater fulfillment and satisfaction. Sex is limited to genitals and intercourse, while sexuality refers to the whole range of attitudes, behaviors, and emotions concerning you and your sexual expression. The book is addressed to men, but women are encouraged to read it as well. Indeed, since sexuality is the most intimate form of human communication, it can be extremely beneficial to a couple's relationship for a woman to gain insight into the needs and conflicts that affect her man.

This book is meant to be comprehensive in covering a wide variety of issues of interest and importance to men. You can read the chapters consecutively, as a survey of male sexuality, or use the book as a reference source to be consulted about specific questions and problems. The book is divided into three sections: chapters on facts to increase your knowledge, chapters on ways to enhance your sexuality, and chapters on dealing with problems that interfere with sexual pleasure. Where there is a question of sexual attitudes and values, I have committed myself to a particular position on the basis of my personal and professional experience as a clinical psychologist and marriage and sex therapist. However, you need to take into account your own background, experiences, and values in deciding how relevant my recommendations are to your own life. In my opinion, the range of normal sexual behavior takes in any private activity between consenting individuals that provides a sense of sharing and pleasure, is not coercive, does not involve children, and is not physically or psychologically destructive. The choice is yours and depends on what you and your partner find satisfying and pleasurable.

A PERSONAL NOTE

My preparation for writing about male sexuality has included not only formal training and study in the field of psychology but also many of the experiences, both negative and positive, that form the typical background of the majority of males in our society. As a boy in Chicago, I received no real sex education from family, church, or school. What knowledge I had came largely from my peers, and if, as a young man, I had taken the sex-myth quiz presented earlier, I would have done poorly. Like most of my friends, I thought of sex primarily in terms of conquest. Although I managed to "score" with a fair number of sex partners, my achievements never seemed quite up to par, and I invariably exaggerated them. I took little responsibility in these early encounters, leaving contraception up to the women. Nor did it occur to me to care about or even notice my partners' responses. When I was twenty-one, I began an affair that lasted for a year and a half, and this was the first time I began to relate to a sex partner on a person-to-person basis—an important learning experience for me.

At the age of twenty-two, I started graduate work in psychology at Southern Illinois University. It was there that I met Emily, and we were married less than a year later. But despite the closeness and affection we felt for each other, I carried with me into the marriage many of the erroneous and destructive assumptions about sex and sex roles that I had learned earlier in my life. This led to problems and conflicts that had to be confronted if we were to achieve emotional and sexual satisfaction in our marriage. Although we never had a sexual dysfunction problem, our sexual relations were only mediocre at first, and it took us well over a year before we became comfortable with sexuality and were able to communicate, experiment, and be spontaneous. Today, after twenty years of marriage and three children (two biological, one adopted), sex continues to be a high-quality, positive part of our marriage. I attribute this not only to the fact that we care deeply about each other but also to the accurate sexual information and positive attitudes we gained through my work in psychology, as a sex and marital therapist, and as a college professor.

My decision to go into the field of sex therapy came about, as such decisions so often do, quite accidentally. I chose a research project in sexual dysfunction and found, to my surprise, that there had been very little work done in that field. This aroused my interst and eventually led me to teaching courses in human sexuality and becoming a sex therapist. I feel that my work as a professional has given me a rather practical viewpoint on sexuality. It seems to me that most sexual Unhappiness is a result of poor learning experiences and a lack of respectful communication between men and women. In many cases, sexual functioning and sexual satisfaction can be improved tremendously, as they were for me, by retracing those early steps to gain a better understanding of one's sexuality and then setting off again with a more aware and positive attitude toward sexuality and toward the woman as a respectful, cooperative, sexual person.

I do not believe that being male is something that one should be ashamed of or apologetic about. Nor do I think that men, either individually or as a group, have to atone for the sins of male chauvinism. No amount of breast-beating can cause relations between a man and woman to become more satisfying. What is needed is not guilt, but understanding, sensitivity, and a commitment to positive change in the present and future. When these are achieved, there is no limit to the pleasure, intimacy, and sense of security that can be derived from a sexual relationship.

In the following chapters I will be dealing with various topics relating to the male sexual life cycle, with methods of enhancing your sexual self-esteem and functioning, with certain decisions and responsibilities that are a necessary part of your sexuality, and dealing with problems that inhibit the full expression of male sexuality. Throughout, I will draw on case studies of clients I have treated (their identities have been disguised), as well as my own personal experiences, to provide relevant illustrations of the points being discussed.

This is basically a book of ideas and information, not a do-it-yourself sex therapy book or a treatise on sexual techniques. If, by presenting an integrated and positive view of male sexuality, my book can help you reexamine your attitudes toward sexuality and regain some of the intimate satisfactions the male performance myths have cheated you out of, I will be satisfied. I hope this book will be helpful to you and the people in your life you care about.

2
THE WORLD'S GREATEST PLEASURE
APPARATUS—YOUR BODY

Almost from the moment we are born, we are fascinated by our bodies. At first it is the mere sensation of having limbs that can extend and contract and thrash about that is an endless source of exhilaration and delight. Later, we learn to coordinate our movements with what we see and discover the distinction between ourselves and the outside world. Within the first year of our development, we find that we can produce enjoyable sensations by rubbing and stroking our genitals: sexual awareness is born. This awareness grows as we mature. Not only is it quite natural for young children to stimulate themselves, but it is also natural for them to be intensely curious about their own sex organs—and those of others around them. Examining and comparing genitals, mutual genital touching, playing "house" or "doctor"—these activities are all a normal part of the process of growing up. These early experiences of looking, touching, and exploring are important in developing attitudes toward oneself, one's body, and sexuality.

Unfortunately, as children, most of us receive strong messages of disapproval that discourage us from pursuing these exploratory practices. We learn that our bodies, and especially our genitals, are something to be hidden, to be ashamed of. Some parents go so far as to teach their children that they should avoid looking at their own bodies. As a result of this negative learning, the natural curiosity we once had about our bodies is blunted. We tell ourselves that the time for self-exploration is over, that we have outgrown such childish pursuits, that there is nothing left to learn. Actually, the average

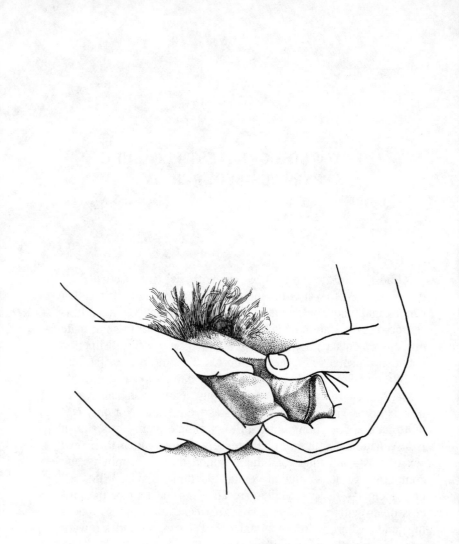

Testicular self-examination

adult knows surprisingly little about his body generally and his genitals specifically. Obeying the dictates laid down by his parents, he imagines that he is acting virtuously by maintaining a state of detached ignorance. Needless to say, such an attitude detracts from a person's capacity to feel comfortable and enjoy his sexuality.

GENITAL EXPLORATION AND AWARENESS

I encourage you to give way to that long-suppressed childhood curiosity and become reacquainted with your body. Find a time when you have at least fifteen or twenty minutes of privacy—it could be the next time you take a bath or shower—and set it aside for sexual self-exploration. Take off your clothes and sit down on the bed or on the floor. A full-length mirror will be helpful because it gives you a more complete view. You may also want to use a hand mirror to look at hard-to-see areas. Relax and, above all, put aside any gnawing thoughts that you are doing something unhealthy. You are only taking a good look at your body, and who has a better right to look at it than you?

Start with the testicles (or balls, if you prefer—you can use proper *or* slang words). Hold them in your hand, using your hand mirror to examine them from all sides. Let yourself become conscious of their weight and shape. You needn't be afraid of hurting them. All of us know from experience how painful a low blow can be, but under normal circumstances, the testicles are surprisingly resilient. Even our dependence on athletic supporters for protection during strenuous activities is largely a learned need. Male animals, whose testicles are no less vulnerable than ours, engage in physical activities that make human athletics seem tame, and yet they suffer no ill effects. Among primitive peoples, males run, dance, and fight without wearing supporters, and they experience no genital injury.

The testicles are the principal male sex glands. Inside the two egg-shaped bodies there are seminiferous tubules, and it is within them that the sperm are manufactured. The testicles also manufacture the male sex hormone, testosterone, which is responsible for triggering the development of male physical characteristics. In combination with psychological factors, testosterone contributes to regulating the sex drive. So efficient are the testicles in maintaining a satisfactory testosterone level that if one of them is removed the remaining testicle is quite capable of carrying on by itself without any decrease in sexual or procreative functioning. If you suspect that your testicles, or any other part of your sexual system, are not functioning properly, the person to see is a urologist. A physician specializing in complaints of the genitourinary tract, the urologist is the closest thing, for men, to a gynecologist. Men are encouraged to do monthly testicle self-examination to insure early detection of testicular cancer (this is similar to the female's self-examination for breast cancer). The male should examine his testicles after a hot bath or shower to determine whether there are small, hard lumps that could be tumors. If you detect anything, you should immediately consult your general physician or a urologist.

Sperm are created by the millions in the testicles. Once they are mature, they leave the testicles by way of the vas deferens, two soft, thin tubes that you can feel going up into the body cavity. The vas leads into the seminal vesicles, storage chambers for the sperm, and then into the prostate. It is in the prostrate that the sperm are mixed with seminal fluid, the whitish, alkaline liquid that spurts from the penis during ejaculation. Sperm are extremely tiny, contributing only slightly to the total volume of the ejaculate, the major portion (95 to 97 percent) of which consists of seminal fluid, or semen. Thus, when the vas deferens is severed in the vasectomy operation, only sperm are left out of the mix. A sterilized male continues to ejaculate seminal fluid as before, with no noticeable decrease in force, amount or enjoyment.

The testicles are housed in a bag of loose, wrinkled skin called the scrotum. In most cases, one testicle, usually the left, hangs lower than the other. The scrotum can contract or relax, at times allowing the testicles to dangle freely against the thighs, at other times drawing them up into a neat, tight package. These changes are brought about, largely in response to a rise or fall in temperature, by tiny muscles in the scrotum. In order to manufacture sperm, the testicles must be a few degrees cooler than body temperature. The scrotum's ability to tighten and loosen is a device for regulating this temperature. When it is cold the muscles contract, warming the testicles by bringing them in close contact with the body. When the outside tempera-

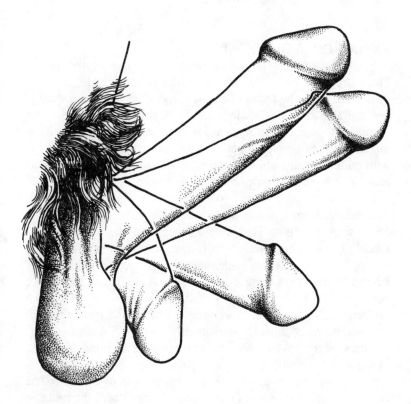

The four states of arousal. Erection is triggered by nerve centers in the lower spinal column signaling blood to enter the penis through arteries running through the erectile tissue.

ture rises, the opposite occurs, and the testicles are repositioned to cool them off.

The scrotal muscles also come into play during sexual excitement. When a man is aroused, his testicles rise in the scrotum and increase in size. If his arousal does not culminate in ejaculation, the swelling remains, causing an uncomfortable condition popularly known as "blue balls." This is temporary, however, and causes no permanent damage.

EXPLORING YOUR PENIS

Emerging just above the scrotum is the base of the penis. There are very few men who have not handled and looked at their penis. It is the focus of intense emotional feelings for men, few are able to regard their penis dispassionately. You may be proud of it, ashamed of it, anxious about it, afraid of it, or have mixed feelings about it, but it is unlikely that you think of it with quite the same attitude you have, for example, toward your ear. Yet the penis is an organ like any other.

It can be an interesting experience to clear your mind of all preconceived notions and to look at your penis as if you have never seen it before. The penis is composed chiefly of spongy erectile tissue. There are, in fact, three distinct cylindrical bodies, two on top and one underneath, which are bound together by sheets of thin membrane. The three cylindrical bodies are what give the penis its somewhat triangular cross section when it is erect. Erection occurs when blood enters the penis through arteries running through the erectile tissue. Simultaneously, muscles near the base of the penis contract, preventing the blood from leaving the penis through the veins. Erection is triggered by nerve centers in the lower spinal column. The actual stimulus that causes erection may come from the brain in the form of erotic thoughts or anticipation, or it may come from direct tactile contact. The first kind of erection, called "spontaneous" or "automatic" erection, is more common in younger men. As men become older, they find that they need more stroking and stimulation of the penis and the genital area in order to obtain an erection. This is not an indication that they are developing an erection problem—erection dysfunction is *not* one of the normal consequences of aging in men—it just means that their pattern of sexual response is changing. The more the man is aware and accepting of his normal bodily changes, the better will be his sexual functioning.

Erection is a natural physiological response. A newborn male baby usually has his first erection within a few minutes of delivery. Every night while sleeping, whether he is currently sexually active or not, the typical male has an erection about every ninety minutes, thus having three to five erections during his night's sleep. Laboratory studies have been done with ninety-year-old men in good health who have been able to get erections and function sexually. You truly are a sexual person from the day you're born to the day you die.

The head of the penis is called the glans. For the majority of males, the glans is the most sensitive part of the penis, having an extremely high concentration of nerve endings. The most sensitive area of the glans is the ridge at its base, called the corona. On the underside of the penis, where the corona divides into a sort of swallowtail shape, there is a small flange of skin joining the glans to the shaft, and it too is frequently highly sensitive. The areas of greatest sensitivity vary according to the individual. Some men, for example, may find that the shaft of their penis is more sensitive than the glans. Some enjoy having their anal area stimulated, while others may find this not at all pleasurable.

In uncircumcised men, the foreskin, or prepuce, extends over the glans but retracts when the penis becomes erect. Jews, Muslims, and many other ethnic and religious groups remove the foreskin in an operation known as circumcision. During the last few decades, circumcision has become a common practice in many advanced nations, but for health reasons rather than religious or cultural ones. The oily substance emitted by the Tyson's glands, located just behind the corona, collects under the uncircumcised foreskin to form a smelly deposit called smegma. Smegma can be eliminated by regular cleanings, but when it is not, it may become a source of infection. Opponents of circumcision have maintained that removal of the foreskin renders a man less sensitive to sexual stimulation and reduces his enjoyment of the sex act. But since it is in the glans and not the foreskin that the concentration of nerve endings is highest, this is untrue. Anyone who feels that his capacity for arousal is not what it should be is wasting time if he tries to pin the blame on his mother's obstetrician.

THE MYTH OF PENIS SIZE

One reason it is particularly important to get our facts straight about male sexual anatomy and physiology is that this area is one that has always been obscured by superstition and misinformation. Men who readily accept scientific findings in other fields will often stubbornly perpetuate myths about the penis as though a loyalty to unsubstantiated sexual folklore is one of the prerequisites of being a "real man." One myth that continues to exert a powerful influence in the face of scientifically established fact concerns penis size. Therefore, in the interest of eliminating the baleful effects of such beliefs, I think it might be beneficial to discuss this particular subject in some detail.

Penis size differences (or imagined differences) have been the basis for an enormous amount of male anxiety. Perhaps the sense of inadequacy has its roots in the childhood experience of a young boy comparing his father's penis with his own. To a child, an adult penis may seem so large and formidable that he can hardly imagine his own organ ever growing to that size. Once such a feeling of inadequacy takes root, it is easily reinforced. One way this commonly occurs is through the practice of making comparisons between one's own penis and those of other males, often in the steamy world of the locker room. What male has not found himself glancing (surreptitiously, of course, so as not to be mistaken for having a homosexual interest) at the genitals of other men as they change into their swimsuits or gym shorts and finding that nearly all of them seem larger than his own?

Actually, such a comparison is misleading for two reasons. First, as the result of perspective, a penis of the same size may look larger when it is seen from a distance as part of someone else's body than when it is seen from above as part of one's own. Second, it is very misleading to judge the size of a penis when it is in the flaccid state. In general, the larger a man's penis when limp, the less it will increase in size when erect. Penises that are smaller in the flaccid state have a greater erectile potential. Thus, there is an equalizing factor in the matter of penis size, and the variations in size among erect penises are much less and are minimally important.

There are individual variations in penis size, of course, just as there are variations in body size. However, penis length varies much less than body height (nor are height and penis size at all related). The average penis is from two and a half to four inches long in the flaccid state and from five and a half to six and a half inches long when erect, with a diameter of about one inch when limp and about one and a half inches when erect. But these are only averages, and, like most averages, they do not mean much, except perhaps that someone, somewhere, has been very busy with a measuring tape. I think it would be far more accurate to say that a normal penis is one that is of proper size to function in intercourse. This definition is one that takes in just about all of us.

The idea that men with larger penises have a stronger sex drive and are capable of greater sexual performance would appear to be a matter of common sense. After all, the larger a man's muscles are, the stronger he usually is. However, as anyone who has taken a course in elementary logic knows, the analogy can be a highly misleading form of reasoning. And the speciousness of this particular idea becomes clear when we examine the results of controlled, scientific testing. Masters and Johnson observed the sexual functioning of hundreds of subjects under laboratory conditions, and they have found no relationship whatever between penis size and sexual desire or functioning.

The related idea that a large penis is capable of giving a woman more pleasure than a small one may be based on the mistaken notion that it is the vagina that is the source of a woman's sexual pleasure. Actually, a woman's most sensitive genital organ is the clitoris—a small, cylindrical organ located at the top of the vestibule at the joining of the labia minora. The clitoris has, in fact, fully as many nerve endings as the glans of the penis, concentrated into a much smaller area. It is the focal point of sexual pleasure in the female, just as the penis is the focal point for the male. During intercourse, the clitoris is stimulated by pulling and rubbing action caused by the couple's pelvic thrusts—a stimulation that is in no way dependent on penis size. The vagina, which is in direct contact with the penis itself, has fewer nerve endings, most of which are in the outer third. Moreover, the vagina is an active rather than passive organ and can adjust to the penis whether it is large or small. The idea of sexual incompatibility based on the size of a couple's sexual organs is, with extremely rare exceptions, a myth.

Because of the distensible nature of the vagina, virtually any man and woman are well suited, at least physically, to give each other pleasure during intercourse. However, as we well know, sexual attraction and functioning are based on much more than genitals.

It must be admitted, of course, that some women may be attracted to men with large penises in much the same way that some men are attracted to women with large breasts. Pornographic films, magazines, and books—with their emphasis on physical endowments—are probably at least partially to blame for encouraging a female obsession with men who are "hung," just as they encourage a male obsession with women who are "stacked." Similarly, they probably reinforce feelings of inadequacy among men and women who think they are not well endowed. But, as we have seen, a woman who imagines that a large penis automatically makes a man an excellent lover is just as naive as a man who believes that all large-breasted women are necessarily easily aroused. A passion for size, on the part of either a man or a woman, may be seen as a preference, and, as such, it is that individual's personal concern. Why should you let someone else's misconceptions serve as a criterion for passing judgment on your own anatomy and sexual self-esteem?

LEARNING TO BE A SEXUAL LOVER

In the last analysis, whatever nature has given us is ours to make the most of. Nor do we have much cause to accuse nature of favoring some men over others. With rare exceptions, we are all about equally suited physically to both give and receive sexual pleasure. Sexual lovers are made, not born. The ability to enjoy sex and to make sex enjoyable for your partner is primarily dependent on the extent of your comfort, skill, sensitivity, imagination, and ability to communicate—all of which are a matter of learning and experience, not natural endowment. Once a man becomes aware of his positive potential as a lover, once he learns how truly satisfying his sex life can be if he gives up performance-oriented sex for pleasure-oriented sex, the question of size can be forgotten.

3
MASTURBATION: THE WAY MEN LEARN TO BE SEXUAL

The traditional manner used to discourage male masturbation is fear and guilt—it will cause blindness, warts, loss of strength, poor sports performance, weakness, erection problems, etc. Fathers have warned sons to avoid "self-abuse" and threatened them with all kinds of punishments, yet the reality is that 95 percent of males masturbate, most of them beginning between the ages of eleven and fifteen. Why? Because it's a normal, healthy part of male sexual development. While most boys and young men admit maturbation feels good, few admit to an unabashed enthusiasm for it. Male adolescents often compare notes on their masturbatory experiences and may at times masturbate together—either in pairs or in groups. But once heterosexual relations become a reality, or even a possibility, masturbation is pushed into the closet. "I don't need it anymore," a young man might say, which is essentially a way of bragging that his sex life is so full that there is simply nothing left over for autoeroticism. But it is only occasionally that such a boast comes anywhere near the truth. The average young, middle-class, unmarried male has intercourse relatively infrequently. Petting to orgasm may account for another, probably somewhat larger, share of his sexual activity. The largest sexual outlet for most adolescent and young adult single men is masturbation; yet, it is only with the utmost reluctance and shame that they are likely to admit this. Married men have an even tougher time confessing the truth. Surveys show that a majority of men continue to masturbate occasionally after marriage. Yet, most men consider masturbation within the marital situation an "abnormality," an indulgence for which there is no justification.

Such an attitude is difficult to understand. Few of us believe anymore that masturbation is physically harmful. Nor would many of us deny that it is pleasurable. Is it not strange then that a harmless pleasure should generate such strong disapproval and guilt feelings?

Actually, it is not strange at all when one considers the prevailing male attitude toward sexuality. For the average male, sex is a goal-oriented activity. The ultimate object is heterosexual intercourse culminating in orgasm; if the man "gives" his partner an orgasm, too, so much the better. Anything else is considered a failure or, perhaps, a mere step on the road to success. Thus, adolescent boys will confront a peer returning from a date with the question "What did you get off her?" "I got tit" is pretty good. "I got two fingers in" is better. But the greatest achievement is, of course, to have had intercourse—to have "scored." The male who has scored the most frequently with the most number of partners is envied by his friends. Clearly, where heterosexual relations are concerned, particularly among young males, quantity is everything, quality practically nothing. The young man who reports to his friends that he and his girlfriend merely caressed each other for an hour but that it was a "fantastic experience" would probably be ridiculed since he failed to "go all the way."

Since intercourse is the male's ultimate sexual goal, it follows that masturbation, which does not contribute directly to the achievement of that goal, serves no practical purpose and, therefore, is unjustified. All that it produces is pleasure, and pleasure, from the traditional male point of view, is not acceptable as an end in itself.

MASTURBATION AND GUILT

Because of the warnings we have been given about masturbation as children, and because of its reputation as a poor substitute for intercourse, most of us feel guilty when we engage in masturbation. This does not stop us from doing it, however. The unfortunate aspect of this situation is not that we are so lacking in self-control, but that our guilt and/or embarrassment prevents us from enjoying masturbation to the fullest and inhibits us from making masturbation the liberating and satisfying experience it can be. When we do masturbate, most of us remain stubbornly goal-oriented. We insist on telling ourselves that these occasional "lapses" serve only one purpose—to relieve sexual tension. Consequently, we get the act over with as quickly as possible—the sooner orgasm is reached, the better. Seldom do we give ourselves the chance to realize that masturbation, far from being a shameful necessity, is actually one of the best ways of learning about our sexual response cycle and of increasing our sensitivity to sexual stimulation—lessons that can then be applied with enormous profit to partner sex.

It may come as a shock to many males for masturbation to be recommended as a positive good. I can almost hear a reader exclaiming, "You're actually telling guys that it's good for them to jerk off?" I am saying just that, but the sort of masturbation I am advocating has little in common with the hurried, goal-oriented, tension-relieving experience so aptly described by terms such as "whacking off," "jerking off," or "beating your meat."

Most males who masturbate bring themselves to orgasm in an average of one to three minutes—often in as little as thirty seconds. The desire to achieve rapid ejaculation originates in early adolescence, with the fear of being caught by a parent or sibling. Most adolescent boys, aware that their parents disapprove of masturbation, develop an understandable reluctance to linger over the experience. They want to get through with it quickly and dispose of the evidence before mom or dad barges in. This pattern is reinforced in the college dormitory situation or group living arrangement where, even though nearly every young man masturbates, none wants the others to know about it. Later on, when a man gains greater privacy, the need for such secrecy disappears, but the habit remains. He takes for his own the negative views of his parents and peers. The male may no longer fear discovery, but he does fear his own loss of self-respect. Hence, he strives to keep the act of masturbation a secret from his conscious mind, cut off from his mature, respectable, day-to-day life.

In a literal sense, he follows the Biblical injunction "Let not thy right hand know what thy left hand doeth." Also, by confining the pleasure to be derived from masturbation to the brief moments of ejaculation, he minimizes his enjoyment of the act, thus appeasing his sense of guilt. My own adolescent masturbatory experiences were the usual ones of hurried and clandestine acts, followed by guilt and embarrassment when I saw semen stains on my sheets.

The exclusive practice of rapid, ejaculation-oriented masturbation can be seen as yet another aspect of the male-machine concept. The male who stimulates his penis with the sole intent of "shooting off" as quickly as possible is, in effect, treating himself like a kind of sexual mechanism. But the penis is not primarily a mechanism. It is an integral part of yourself, a part of the enormously complex pattern of interacting physical and psychological components that make you a human being.

Nor is your penis the only part of you that is sexual. It does have a very high concentration of nerve endings. But then so do other parts of your body, such as your hands, thighs, and face. And as anyone knows who has ever had a massage, parts of the body whose nerve counts are relatively low, such as the back, can be extremely susceptible to pleasurable sensations. What I am saying is that your whole body is a sex organ. Your mind is your major sex organ, with your penis being a distant second. Masturbation need not be only a way of triggering brief, intense sensations localized in the penis. It can be a method of awakening the sexual potential of the entire body. As such, it can serve to vastly increase a man's capacity for sexual awareness, which is good in and of itself as well as being valuable for partner sex.

ALLOWING YOURSELF TO EXPERIENCE MASTURBATION

The slower, sensuous, whole-body masturbation that I am recommending and that I will describe in detail may be somewhat threatening to many men. In order to assuage their guilt feelings, men tell themselves that they don't masturbate for sexual and erotic sensations, but solely to relieve tension. There can be no doubt, though, that when you masturbate more slowly, concentrating on the pleasure you are experiencing, what you are doing is erotic. This may be disturbing at first. You may be afraid that thoughts and feelings you find uncomfortable and strange might emerge and take control. In fact, sensuously oriented masturbation can show you parts of yourself of which you were unaware. But you needn't fear such revelations. Just as it is a truism that in order to accept love from others you must learn to respect and value yourself, it is also true that in order to accept and feel comfortable with sexual stimulation from a partner you must learn to experience the pleasure and responsiveness of your own body.

The concept that most of us have of our own sexuality is unnecessarily rigid. The fact that you can respond to your body does not make you a narcissist. Quite the contrary, a man's failure to be a responsive, imaginative lover can often be ascribed to the fact that he is not in touch with his own body. By developing the capacity to experience a greater range of pleasure and sensuality, we are likely to derive more pleasure from our bodies through self-stimulation than we thought possible. Equally important, our heightened self-awareness will make us more conscious of our partner's sexual needs and responses. Before we can guide and direct our partners in the kind of touching and pleasuring that are most arousing for us, we need to discover and accept this stimulation from ourselves. A sexually aware man is one who is knowledgeable about and responsible for his own sexuality, and who can interact sensitively with a partner. Thus, masturbation can serve to enhance your masculinity.

Arthur

Arthur, a client of mine, provides a good example of how different mechanically oriented masturbation and sensuous masturbation can be in their effect on a man's sex life. A reporter for a large city newspaper, thirty-seven, and divorced, Arthur had a twenty-year history of premature ejaculation that was related to his general anxiety about sex. Ever since adolescence, Arthur had masturbated rapidly and furtively. His only remembrance of his father telling him anything about sex was when father said, "If I ever catch you playing with yourself, I'll beat you silly!" That didn't stop Arthur from masturbating, but it did increase his sense of guilt and anxiety, as well as the rapidity of his response.

In his sexual experience with women, Arthur always ejaculated quickly. Arthur had very little understanding or appreciation of affectionate touching or sensual pleasuring. He came to me for help in overcoming his rapid ejaculation problem so he could have greater confidence in starting a new relationship with a woman. As part of his therapy, I had him engage in prolonged sensuous touching and self-exploration, but without going to orgasm. He was uncomfortable doing this the first time and said he felt silly stopping before he ejaculated. But the second time was better and the third better still. After three weeks, Arthur was able to stimulate himself for a prolonged period of time and reach a high level of arousal while maintaining voluntary control over ejaculation. He learned that the process of getting there was enjoyable. He was able to stimulate himself for between ten and fifteen minutes before coming to orgasm. When he was orgasmic he found it more pleasurable and satisfying than before. This masturbatory experience helped him overcome his rapid ejaculation problem with a partner.

GUIDELINES FOR SENSUOUS MASTURBATION

Although it is usual for masturbation to end with orgasm, try to rid yourself of the preconception that each masturbation experience *must* end in orgasm. Remember, we are trying to get away from the male-machine concept of the body. Try not to think of your genitals as a mechanism that must be forced to react in a certain predictable way. Rather concentrate on stimulating your genitals, as well as the rest of your body, in various ways and observe your responses. Resist the temptation to judge a particular feeling as either bad or good according to whether it produces a strong erection or hastens ejaculation. There is no disputing the fact that, in terms of the intensity of pleasure, ejaculation is the high point of any male sexual experience. However, in order to broaden and deepen our capacity for erotic response, we should be able to occasionally forego the high point for the sake of exploring the range of our sensual feelings. Try not to become anxious if a particular stimulus does not bring you closer to orgasm. To a certain extent, we are all ejaculation addicts, and there is a tendency, when slow, whole-body stimulation is not producing a strong response, to say, "Forget this nonsense, let's get down to business with some good old-fashioned pumping." If you do get frustrated and move quickly to orgasm don't put yourself down. There's always a next time. But remember, just because you are not responding strongly at the moment does not mean that you have lost your capacity to respond. The ejaculation is there when you want it. So relax and enjoy yourself.

Second, most of us, even those who consider themselves liberal or flexible in other areas, are arch-conservatives when it comes to masturbation techniques. A man who orders roast beef and baked potato every time he eats in a restaurant would be considered pretty unadventurous. But this is exactly what most of us do when we masturbate. The average male works out a certain technique for masturbation during early adolescence, and thereafter he sticks to that technique until the day when his penis and hand finally part company, convinced all the while that his is the only technique possible. It may surprise such diehards to learn that there are virtually as many masturbation techniques as there are masturbators. Masters and Johnson, who studied masturbation in a laboratory setting, found that no two of their subjects used precisely the same method. And yet it rarely occurs to most of us to vary the technique we've become accustomed to. Again, we seem determined not to try to increase the pleasure we derive from masturbation. Just as experimentation is to be encouraged in lovemaking, it is also to be encouraged in masturbation.

Finally, a few words about how to deal with anxiety. You may find that some of the exercises cause you to feel uncomfortable. This is quite understandable. After all, the habits of a lifetime are not broken easily. The important thing to remember is that if you feel anxious or uncomfortable as a result of touching yourself in a particular place or in a particular way, don't stop, but go back to an earlier movement, one that caused you no anxiety. Or if you do stop for a while—do so with the intention to return to the exercise when the anxiety dissipates. In this way, you will be able to carry out your self-exploration in slow, easy stages rather than give in to the anxiety and go back to your rigid system. Your goal is not to reach orgasm, but rather to explore your body. Remember, you are doing this for yourself. You deserve to be treated gently and with respect. Any masturbation technique, as long as it's not physically harmful or compulsive, is in the normal range.

SELF-EXPLORATION/MASTURBATION EXERCISES

As adolescents we masturbate in response to sexual tension, usually without much thought about how we do it. The hand moves to the penis without conscious thought, the movements follow the well-worn tracks of a habitual pattern. There is nothing wrong with masturbation of this sort, but it serves no purpose other than providing simple, uncomplicated climax, easing mental or physical stress. Like most habits, it moves only in a tight, unvarying circle of desire and reward, going nowhere. In fact, for many men masturbation is a response to anxiety, rather than a pleasurable experience. I encourage such men to masturbate only when they are ''horny'' or want a sex outlet, and not to masturbate when they feel anxious. There are psychologically healthier ways to deal with anxiety than masturbation.

Exercise 1. In order to make masturbation a learning experience, we must vary the pattern. Relaxation of the body and mind is essential in setting the stage for such an experience. A leisurely bath or shower is a good way to begin. As you wash yourself, using scented soap if you like, massage your arms, shoulders, back and legs. You probably have an inner timing device that goes off in your head when you think your allotted time in the tub has expired. Ignore it. Give yourself permission to stay until you feel relaxed and refreshed and ready for the next phase. Be conscious of your sensations as you move from a wet environment to a dry one—the dripping of water from your body, the slight chill if it is cool, the breaking out of tiny, clean beads of sweat if it is hot. Dry yourself vigorously, concentrating on the feel of the rough towel on your skin.

Without putting on your clothes, go into the bedroom and make whatever preparations you need to feel comfortable. This may include turning down the lights, putting on music, turning on the air conditioner. Lie down on the bed in an unrestrained position. Luxuriate. Enjoy your sense of physical freedom. Remember, there is no one watching you or judging how you look. You can achieve a state of relaxation by tensing the muscles in each part of your body in succession, then focusing on the feeling as you release the tension. Breathe slowly, deeply, and evenly, repeating the word *relax* to yourself in rhythm with your breathing.

When you are relaxed, roll over on your side, focusing on the way your body feels as you move. Touch yourself slowly and gently, avoiding the genital areas at this point. You might try closing your eyes at first, so you can focus better on your sensations. Move from feet to head, noticing how each part of your body feels when you touch it. Vary the pressure of your touching from light to heavy, noticing your response to different types of touch.

After you feel you have explored your body sufficiently through touch, you may want to turn to visual exploration. Get up and look at yourself in a full-length mirror. Try to see your body objectively, the way you might look at a piece of sculpture. Instead of making judgments about yourelf, such as "I'm too fat" or "My chest is too flabby," concentrate on the curves and masses of the different parts of your body, noticing the way they fit together. You could use a second mirror to view your body from the rear. Look at yourself in a way you have never done before, such as standing with your back to the mirror, bending over, and looking at your reflection through your legs.

Now concentrate on your genitals. Examine our penis, looking at and touching its various parts, including the glans, corona, and shaft. Examine your scrotum and testicles. Notice how your genitals look when you stand up, sit down, and lie down. The idea of this exploration is to help you to feel comfortable with your body. When you feel that you have achieved this objective—and this may take from one to several sessions—you can move on to the second exercise.

Exercise 2. Prepare for the second exercise with a leisurely shower or bath, followed by a few minutes of deep breathing and muscle relaxation. This time, concentrate more on specifically erotic sensations. Touch yourself in whatever way you find most sensually pleasing. Try stimulating your nipples, which can be highly sensitive in many men, just as they are in women. Notice how they become erect after stroking or massage.

Taking your time, begin stroking the insides of your thighs. Run your fingers through your pubic hair, noticing the sensations that occur when you do so. Finally move your hand to your penis. Experiment with different types of touching and stroking to discover the method you find most arousing. Try a technique of penile stimulation that you do not ordinarily use. If you usually use hard strokes, try gentle ones. If you are accustomed to stimulating only the shaft of your penis, concentrate on the glans. Experiment with stroking and holding the testicles as well, using your other hand. You may continue this stimulation until you reach orgasm, but do not feel under any pressure to do so. The object of this exercise is to help you to acquire new knowledge of and comfort with genital stimulation.

Exercise 3. This time omit or include the preliminary shower, whichever you prefer. Bathing is a sensual and relaxing experience, but there is no need to make a ritual of it. Concentrate initially on nongenital touching and caressing, noticing which sorts of stimulation are most rewarding for you. You may wish to experiment with erotic literature or pictures as a device for enhancing arousal. Fantasies are used by the great majority of males during masturbation, so feel free to use written or pictorial material to enhance the masturbatory experience. Do not fall into the trap of opting for rapid, genital-oriented stimulation to orgasm, but be aware, as your arousal slowly mounts, of the complete cycle of sexual stimulation. Notice how your penis becomes larger and harder as ejaculation approaches, how the glans swells and becomes suffused with blood. Be aware of the increasing muscle tension in your body.

Just before you begin to ejaculate, notice the intensely positive sensations at the point of ejaculatory inevitability, when orgasm is no longer a voluntary response. When you do begin ejaculating one to three seconds later, concentrate on those moments of intense sensation. Feel the contractions of the ejaculatory ducts within the penis, look at the semen as it spurts from the penis. After ejaculation has ended, notice how your penis loses its erectness. Also notice how your breathing and heartbeat have speeded up during arousal and are now returning to normal levels. Do you feel sleepy or energetic after an orgasm? Examine your semen, noticing the way it feels and smells. Try to become accustomed to it and comfortable with it. You may even want to put a drop on your tongue to see how it tastes. The object of this exercise is to help you accept and appreciate the natural and total functioning of your body during sexual arousal.

Exercise 4. In this last exercise, continue your experimentation to find the kinds of stimulation that are most arousing for you. Introduce one or more elements into this exercise that you have not tried before. You may, for example, wish to experiment with some lubricant such as a lotion, oil, or cream. Or try masturbating by lying facedown and rubbing your penis against the sheet or pillow. You might try rolling a towel into a cylinder and inserting your penis inside to simulate a vagina. Include the nongenital touching you've learned to enjoy. Feel free to use any fantasy or erotic material as mental stimulation. Don't restrict yourself, and fully enjoy the process of bringing yourself to orgasm. Celebrate the full extent of your capacity for arousal.

THE POSITIVE ROLE OF MASTURBATION

After completing these exercises, it should be clear to you that masturbation, far from being a "poor excuse for the real thing," can be a rewarding sexual experience in its own right. Learning to use masturbation to gain pleasure and self-knowledge rather than just as a penis-oriented sexual safety valve is an excellent way of becoming comfortable with your body and its natural and healthy responsiveness to stimulation. It is amazing how, once you begin to try sensuous, whole-body self-stimulation, the pleasure of the experience—no longer confined to the brief three to ten seconds of orgasm—expands into a whole new world of erotic sensations. Not only is this very pleasurable in itself, but it can help you to respond more effectively with your partner during foreplay/pleasuring, intercourse and during afterplay/afterglow.

4

SEX AND THE UNMARRIED MALE

Until the 1960s, sex among the unmarried in our society was unofficially regulated by the sexual double standard. Unmarried men and unmarried women were expected to conform to quite different codes of conduct. For an adolescent boy, gaining premarital sexual experience was a goal to be sought as part of his rite of passage to manhood. Virginity was an embarrassment, a mark of shame. No adolescent male over sixteen would admit to being a virgin (although the majority were). The young man who "scored" with the greatest number of women was an object of envy and admiration to his peers. The adolescent female, on the other hand, was taught that her sexuality was a valuable possession to be protected—saved in a hope chest, as it were—until it could be bestowed untarnished on a husband (or at least a fiancé). The limits of acceptable female sexual behavior varied from family to family and from community to community, but one rule remained constant: unmarried women were not supposed to "go all the way." They were expected to remain virgins until they married, or to have premarital sex only with the male they planned to marry.

PRESSURE ON WOMEN
This double standard created an interesting dilemma. If young men were expected to become sexually experienced before marriage while young women were not, with whom then were the young men supposed to acquire their experience? The solution to this problem depended on the existence of two different classes

32

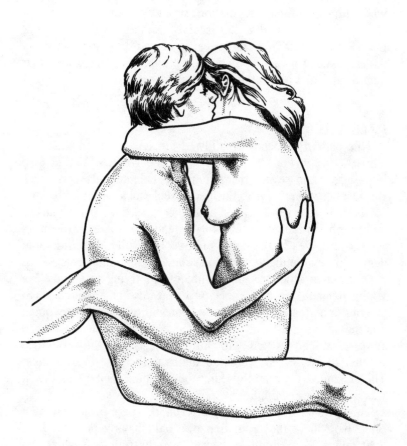

Today's best indications suggest that about 90% of men and 80% of women have sex prior to marriage.

of unmarried women—"good girls" and "bad girls." Good
girls were, of course, the ones who followed society's dictates
and were virginal. Bad girls were the ones who gave in—who
had intercourse and thereby "cheapened" themselves. In actual-
ity, this distinction was not so strictly maintained. Not every
girl who had sex before marriage become "bad." It was only
when a girl acquired a reputation, when she began to be known
for being "easy," that her social standing was threatened.
Interestingly, this was the reverse of the situation faced by
males; a young man's reputation for promiscuity enhanced rather
than diminished his status.

PRESSURE ON MEN

This pattern of behavior allowed greater sexual freedom for
unmarried men than it did for unmarried women. Yet, it also
imposed certain severe restrictions on male sexual expression.
Because "scoring" was considered such an indispensable sign
of masculinity, sex became highly competitive, performance-
and number-oriented. There was a tendency to see women as
objects, trophies in the game of sexual pursuit. A considerable
degree of manipulativeness was condoned in the behavior of
a young man who was in the process of trying to "make" a
young woman. He was expected to be false and seductive, to
pretend to a greater intimacy or responsibility toward the woman
than he actually felt—all in the interest of getting her to "come
across" and go to bed with him. Male "lines" to convince
women to be sexual were the material for jokes and books.
They changed with the fads, but the common theme was that it
was a game, a manipulation.

This persistent pushing for sex on the part of young men
often won them the reputation of "only having one thing on
their minds"—meaning, of course, sex. In truth, it was not just
the sexual experience that spurred them on in their efforts;
rather, it was the glory of having had sex, that great initiating
experience that was so crucial in confirming the manhood of an
adolescent male. Sex as status, sex as accomplishment—these
were of major importance in motivating a young male to seek
out sexual liaisons. Real sexual feelings played a part in these
encounters, too, of course. But the quality of the experience

itself was overlooked or viewed as unimportant. The real emphasis was on competition among the young men. As in poker, bluffing was a legitimate tactic in this sexual game, and a young man would fabricate or exaggerate his own exploits in order to advance himself in the eyes of his peers. This set the stage for the male pattern that extends throughout the life span—brag and "one up" each other about sex, never admit problems or ask questions, and be the self-contained expert.

Most young men were so caught up in this pursuit of conquest that much of the pleasure was lost. Premarital sex was surrounded by such negative societal sanctions that young people, both male and female, were too anxious and ill at ease to enjoy the actual experience in anything remotely approaching its full potentiality. The trouble was that the double standard not only imposed to separate codes of behavior on men and women, but that it made them rather ill suited as sex partners as well. Both tended to identify far too strongly with stereotyped role models—that is, men were expected to be aggressive and women passive. Thus, whole areas of experience and pleasure were effectively closed off to both sexes. Males tended to be eager for sex, willing to try out variations in sexual behavior, relatively uninhibited sexually. On the other hand, they seemed to have an incapacity for tenderness and warmth, as well as an inability to integrate their emotions with the physical expression of sexuality. For males, *sex* meant "intercourse." If there was only affection and pleasuring, the woman had gotten the best of him and he labeled her a "cock teaser." Women tended to be less enthusiastic about sex, less adventurous, and more afraid of their own sexuality. Yet, they did seem to be more open and responsive in interpersonal relationships, and to have a greater appreciation for affection and sensuality.

MOVING AWAY FROM THE DOUBLE STANDARD

During the past two decades, there have been major changes in our attitudes toward sexuality in general, with much of this change focused upon premarital sex. The restrictive double standard is no longer dominant in contemporary society. There is a growing movement for women to step out of their passive role and to be active and involved sexually. The old sanctions against premarital sex have broken down, and it is now the norm of unmarried men and women to have sex. Premarital sexual experience no longer brands a young woman as "bad." In fact, being a virgin can now be as much of a burden to a woman as it is to a man. There has been a moderate change in the incident of premarital sex for men during the past decade, and a more substantial, although hardly revolutionary, change for women. Previously, about 80 percent of males had intercourse before marriage, as compared to approximately 50 percent of females. At present, best indications are that the figures are approximately 90 percent for males and 80 percent for females. The older the person is at marriage (and the average age is now twenty-five for males and twenty-three for females), the more likely he or she is to have had premarital intercourse. The average age for the first intercourse experience is now seventeen for males and nineteen for females. While it is true that the old double standard may be on its way out, there is some question as to whether the system that is replacing it is much of an improvement, in terms of an emotionally integrated and rewarding approach to sexuality.

The new sexual attitudes too often seem to require that both men and women live up to the aggressive, competitive standards that used to apply exclusively to men, and there is a danger that women as well as men are giving more importance to performance than to pleasure. This was ironically demonstrated when Masters and Johnson published their material on female multiple orgasm. Suddenly a new performance demand had come into existence, a new standard against which to measure sexual ability. Many women who considered themselves sexually liberated began to feel anxious if they had never been multiorgasmic (less than one in five adult women are multi-orgasmic, and the numbers are even lower for adolescent and young adult women). Current studies indicate that this new performance anxiety may manifest itself in the form of sexual dysfunction. There is an increase in women who have been orgasmic and are now nonorgasmic, very possibly as a result of their attempts to become multiorgasmic, or have "G" spot orgasms, or whatever is the current faddish performance criterion. How unfortunate it would be if the old double standard was being replaced by a new code of behavior that was coercive—in terms of exerting pressure to meet a particular standard of performance—rather than genuinely liberating.

PUTTING PREMARITAL SEX IN PERSPECTIVE

Part of the problem is that premarital sex has been given too much attention. Whether premarital sex is forced underground by societal sanctions as it was in the past, or celebrated and ballyhooed in the media as it is today, the result is essentially the same: premarital sex is overemphasized at the expense of mature adult sexuality. According to contemporary stereotypes, sex that takes place primarily between unmarried people in their teens and twenties is seen as glamorous, tantalizing, and rather explosive. The emphasis on premarital sex as premarital intercourse downplays the range of sexual expression. Sex as an intimate sharing of pleasure between an adult couple who are deeply committed to one another has been largely ignored. Whether they are operating under the old, repressive double standard or under the newer, coercive single standard, young people feel entirely too pressured to "prove" themselves sexually. Perhaps we ought to cease focusing on questions such as "Should they or shouldn't they?" and look at premarital sex from the prespective of a person's lifetime involvement with sexuality. Instead of seeing the premarital phase as a time of intense sexual activity—a sort of sexual proving ground—we should regard it as an initial explorative foray into the world of adult sexuality, a kind of apprenticeship.

A MORE POSITIVE APPROACH TO
PREMARITAL SEXUALITY

A more honest, nonmanipulative single standard of premarital sexuality needs to be developed—one that would combine the stereotypical man's eagerness for sexual expression and the woman's interest in relationships and feelings. Rather than the woman copying the man in being sexually manipulative and exploitative, she would allow herself to be sexually expressive and comfortable in the context of a respectful, communicative, nonmanipulative relationship. In turn, the man would learn to accept his sexuality as a means of expressing and sharing intimate feelings and of giving and receiving pleasure, rather than as an inherently self-centered demand to be satisfied through exploitation. Perhaps the most necessary adjustment for a young man to make is to see the woman as a sexual person rather than an object. A sexual object can be manipulated, used, and eventually discarded. But if seen as a sexual person, a woman becomes someone whose needs, both physical and personal, must be considered and dealt with. What I am advocating is a more honest and respectful relationship between the sexes. Both men and women must be willing to change and to learn, and the best time for this learning process to begin is at the outset of a person's sexual career—during the premarital years.

A young man who is accustomed to being manipulative in sex, who has treated his sex partners as objects—as prizes to be acquired—and who has had little practice in communicating honestly with women, will find it difficult to change after he gets married. Nor do women automatically blossom sexually when they marry. Rather, if their premarital learning stressed that they were not to engage in sex too freely or enthusiastically, this attitude is likely to linger. Thus, the old double standard is an unpromising basis for a marital relationship.

The negative effects of the double standard on women have been emphasized, and rightly so. The woman is discouraged from developing an aware, responsible, affirmative view of her sexuality, and this inhibits adult sexual expression. Yet, it is becoming clearer that in the long run it is the male who experiences more negative effects from the double standard. The adult male finds it quite difficult to integrate emotional feelings and sexual expression into a genuinely intimate marital relationship. Even more, he finds it hard to view his wife as his equal partner and sexual friend. Males learn to be sexual outside the context of a giving relationship. The young man is able to experience desire, arousal, and orgasm without needing anything from his partner. As he becomes thirty and older, he needs a more cooperative, giving relationship to function and enjoy sex. His premarital training inhibits his being able to ask for, much less engage in, such a relationship. Nor is it a help if both partners are influenced by the newer, false, single standard in which both men and women are expected to conform to the aggressive, competitive standards that once governed the sexual behavior of males. Thus, for the sake of achieving fulfillment in adult life, as well as for the sake of present satisfaction, it is important that young men (and women) establish guidelines for making decisions about their premarital behavior that will allow them to feel good about their sexuality.

One of the basic difficulties of premarital sex is the question of whom to choose as a partner. In the past, the double standard of behavior made it quite clear just what was expected of young people. But now that it has become generally acceptable for both men and women to express themselves sexually, new issues have arisen. In a society where the choice of behavior is left largely up to the individual, the burden of making decisions that accord with your personal value system becomes far greater. We no longer have the clear dos and don'ts of society to fall back upon. The double standard was understood, but wrong. The new premarital standards are very confusing and unclear. The predominant premarital standard of sex with affection is more psychologically reasonable, but complex and difficult to put into practice. In a sense, we are like children whose mother has given us free run of the cookie jar; the question has suddenly changed from "How many cookies can I get?" to "How many and what kind of cookies do I want?" Are we obligated to prove the vigor of our appetites by gobbling as many as we can get our hands on? The problem is harder for males because they have been schooled in the doctrine that a real man never turns down an opportunity to have sex. Thus, it is particularly important for us to establish some basic guidelines for managing our sexual relationships.

CIRCLES OF INTIMACY

We might start by examining our normal social life. If we think about the people whose lives touch on our own, it becomes apparent that we are involved with many people on several different levels, and that these involvements can be categorized according to the degree of intimacy they entail. Human relationships are, of course, highly complex, and any attempt to fit them into categories is arbitrary. Nevertheless, it is worthwhile trying, since by doing so we gain a certain clarity and perspective on interpersonal relationships generally, and sexual relationships specifically.

The average person's relationships can be seen as fitting into five categories. We may visualize these categories as a series of concentric circles. The closer to the center, the more intimacy involved; the larger the circle, the less intimacy involved. As the relationship becomes closer, the degree of trust, caring, and emotional involvement increases, but so also does the individual's vulnerability to being hurt.

In circle E—the outermost circle—are all those people whose lives intersect with yours in some way, but about whom you know virtually nothing, somtimes not even their names. This group, whose number is potentially unlimited, might include a clerk in a store, a bus driver, a receptionist in an office, people you pass in the street. Your interaction with them is purely coincidental and involves no degree of intimacy at all. The next circle, D, contains those people with whom you may have established a certain elementary degree of contact, but no real personal involvement—people you may see on a regular basis and chat with occasionally about relatively neutral topics. You may know their names and some facts about them, but if they were to suddenly disappear from your life, you would experience little emotional reaction. At any given time there could be a hundred or more people like this in your life, and during the course of your lifetime, perhaps thousands.

Relationships that involve a degree of real intimacy begin with circle C. These are people you refer to as friends, people with whom you have shared some of your feelings and whose attitude toward you is a matter of some concern. You care about these people, and if they were to disappear from your life, a definite emotional gap would be created, although not a devastating one. Circle C friends are those who fade out of your life as circumstances change—you move, a job change, etc. The average person may have five to fifteen such friends at any given time, and probably more than a hundred in the course of a lifetime.

Circle B includes close friends, people who know a great deal about you and who you trust enough to divulge your intimate feelings. The average person may have one, two, or three such friends at any given time and perhaps ten to twenty-five during his life. These are people you try to maintain contact with even if your life circumstances change. Circle B close friendships are an important, ongoing part of your life and contribute to your self-esteem and feelings of belonging in the world. When a close relationship of this sort comes to an end, there is usually a feeling of sadness and hurt.

Circle A includes only very close, intimate relationships such as one has with a best friend, a lover, a spouse, or an adult who serves as a mentor or confidant. These relationships involve a sense of deep commitment as well as emotional intimacy. We allow people in circle A to know our innermost thoughts, to gain an awareness of our personal strengths and weaknesses. These are people we trust and care about and we really expect them to ''be there'' for us. When a circle A relationship ends, we are affected profoundly, experiencing a deep sense of loss. In one's whole life there are usually no more than seven to ten circle A relationships, and for many people there may be as few as one or two.

We can use this circles-of-intimacy concept to examine the values that serve as a basis for making decisions about our sexual relationships. According to the old double standard (which assumed that a man should be willing and able to have sex with any woman, anytime, anywhere), a woman from any of the circles would be a potential sexual partner. On the other hand, a woman would be expected to have sex only with a man occupying circle A—namely her husband or her fiancé. The double standard required a man to utilize deception and manipulation in his attempt to convince a potential partner that his feelings went much deeper than they really did, that his level of caring and emotional involvement approached that of circle A.

But such behavior is poor preparation for a mature relationship. Thus, it is to our advantage to try to be honest and clear about which circle of intimacy a particular woman who attracts us occupies. This does not necessarily mean that we can only have sex with women from circles A and B. What it does mean is that we should not enter into a sexual encounter under false pretenses. For example, it could be acceptable for a man and woman whose degree of intimacy placed them only within circle D to have sex, provided they both knew just where they stood with respect to one another. If, on the other hand, the woman was dissatisfied with a circle D relationship and wished for a degree of intimacy characterized by circle B, it would be unacceptable for the man to pretend that such a relationship existed merely to have sex with her. This circles-of-intimacy concept is equally applicable to women, and thus could prove useful in moving us closer to a single standard of premarital sexual expression. This would provide a better basis for adult sexual functioning for men and women alike.

There is nothing inherently wrong with casual sex, so long as the participants have no illusions about it and they practice safe sex in terms of contraception and diseases. However, sex is generally more satisfying when a degree of intimacy exists between the partners. For one thing, it is easier in a more intimate, trusting relationship to be honest about your sexual preferences and responses, and this communication will mean increased sexual satisfaction. Assuming that you are interested in enhancing the quality of your sex life, you would probably do well to limit your choice of partners to people from circle C or closer. Since circles C, B, and A are likely to contain no more than fifteen to twenty individuals at any given time, such a decision goes a long way toward simplifying your sexual involvements. This guideline applies equally well to homosexual and heterosexual relationships. Trust and intimacy are just as important in a sexual relationship between two members of the same set as they are between a man and a woman.

Using the circles-of-intimacy concept to plan and order your sex life may at first seem to be a strange idea. Most of us tend to think that sex should be a spontaneous occurrence and that deliberately planning your sexual activity would make it less enjoyable. Actually, planning can often make real spontaneity possible, for it can help you avoid problems—diseases or unwanted pregnancy, for example—as well as increase feelings of comfort and self-confidence. The basic point to remember is that sexuality is an integral part of you as a person and should enhance your life rather than cause difficulties.

FIRST INTERCOURSE

Nowhere is planning more needed—yet nowhere is it more often avoided—than in first intercourse experiences. Because it is usually so significant for a male, whether it occurs at age fifteen or thirty-five, the first intercourse would ideally be planned, adequate contraceptive measures would be utilized, and it would occur in a nondemanding situation. The experience would be further enhanced if the couple was comfortable with each other and had at least once or twice engaged in relaxed pleasuring activities before attempting intercourse. This crucial first experience should be seen not as a performance but as a natural event arising out of increased intimacy and arousal.

Unfortunately, few (if any) men undergo their sexual initiation in such ideal circumstances. Typically, first intercourse experiences are characterized by intense anxiety based partly on the fear of failure and partly on the fear of being caught in the act. Only about one out of three first-time couples use some form of contraception. The contraceptive device used most frequently is the condom, and it is generally put on in a hurried and clumsy manner. Since first intercourse is usually a time of high anxiety and low skill, it is surprising when it goes well at all. About 25 percent of males experience failure due to an inability to get or maintain an erection or because they ejaculate before the penis enters the vagina. The great majority of men ejaculate quickly during their first intercourse. It is important, therefore, not to overreact to an unsuccessful or unenjoyable first intercourse experience. Be aware that sexual enjoyment takes practice and cooperation. Above all, it is essential to remember that the human male is not a sexual machine that can be expected to function flawlessly whenever the button of sexual stimulation is pressed.

PREMARITAL SEXUALITY AS A LEARNING EXPERIENCE

If a young man is able to think of premarital sex not as a "proving ground" but rather as a learning opportunity, a time of apprenticeship for the long period of mature sexuality to come, much of the pressure of permarital sexuality will be diminished. The less one thinks of sex as a performance and the more one thinks of it as a personally fulfilling and enhancing experience, the more enjoyable it will be. Once we are able to accustom ourselves to the fact that we are still at a learning stage and that we are not alone in this, we can become more accepting of our own mistakes, confident that we are benefiting from these early experiences and that they will contribute to our later sexual adjustment. There is a joy to learning about any field, and there is no reason for sex to be an exception.

There is a feeling of satisfaction in knowing that, from one relationship to the next, you are learning to overcome hang-ups, communicate more effectively, make love more skillfully and sensitively, and treat your sex partner as a person. You also have to realize that some sexual relationships might be mistakes that will cause pain and leave a bad feeling. These negative occurrences can also serve as learning experiences. The real value of premarital sex is not in proving yourself a sexual superman but in feeling that you are growing as a person and learning to make your sexuality a positive force in your life as well as integrating it more fully with your emotions.

The percentage of men who succeed in making such an adjustment is still not great, but there are enough of them around to hope that comfortable, pleasurable, and learning-oriented premarital sex is the wave of the future.

Jon

Jon is one such example. A twenty-four-year-old graduate student who works as a trainee for a communications company, Jon enjoys his job, likes to travel, and is generally pleased with his sex life. He did not have intercourse until he was nineteen and was somewhat concerned at the time that he was lagging behind his friends, but gave up these fears when he became sexually active. Most of his affairs have tended to be fairly intimate ones. He has had four sex partners in about the same number of years. He felt little pressure to "score" with a greater number of women merely for the sake of achieving prestige among his male friends. In his first affair, neither Jon nor his partner used any form of contraception, and there were two rather disturbing pregnancy scares. Since then, he has been careful about preventing unwanted pregnancy and uses a condom when his partner is not using the pill, an IUD, or a diaphragm. More recently, Jon has had sexual relationships of shorter duration—two one-night stands and two affairs lasting for only a few weeks. From these experiences he has learned that he enjoys himself more, both personally and sexually, when he feels a genuine sense of companionship with the woman. He has also discovered that the more he likes a woman on a personal basis, the more he will want to engage in a wider range of sexual acts, such as fellatio and cunnilingus, with her. Moreover, he finds that his own pleasure is enhanced when a woman is responsive and really enjoys the sexual experience with him. Jon does not think he will marry until he is in his late twenties, and he is looking forward to continuing to enjoy sex as a single man in the interim period. He does not view marriage as a comedown from premarital sex, but as an opportunity to use the sexual knowledge and skill he has acquired to develop and sustain a long-term, intimate, committed relationship. I predict great success for him.

CLOSING THOUGHTS

Perhaps not everyone can be as fortunate as Jon in managing premarital sex. Adolescence and young adulthood are often confusing and conflict-filled times when negative experiences of one kind or another are almost certain to occur. But if you remember that satisfying sexual relations require comfort, and that sexual experiences that do not go well can be used as learning opportunities, you will have made important progress in achieving a good sexual adjustment. The young man, in accepting responsibility for his sexuality, needs to learn not only to value experimentation and to be comfortable with different techniques but also to communicate his feelings and to enjoy intimacy. This will lead to the development of a genuine single standard of premarital behavior that will be beneficial for both men and women, and more important, will promote sexual satisfaction in adulthood.

5
CONTRACEPTION: PLEASURE, NOT PATERNITY

We usually conceptualize sex as a means of intimate communication, a sharing of pleasure. And certainly, for men and women today, this aspect is by far the most important one. But there is, of course, another aspect that we must come to terms with, because its influence is extremely important. I am referring to sex as a means of reproduction.

People have historically believed that reproduction is the purpose of sex. Sexual pleasure, then, is the prize that nature offers us for multiplying our kind. If this prize did not exist, if each couple had to go about reproducing itself in a wholly rational, deliberate, and nonpleasurable way, it is unlikely that the human race would have grown to its present population.

Sex accomplishes the task of preserving the human race much too well, however. In our advanced society, where widely available medical facilities insure that nearly all children will survive to reproductive age themselves, the biological function of sex presents a serious problem. Couples who pursue the prize of sexual pleasure without thought for the consequences are likely to find themselves with more offspring than they can afford to house, clothe, and feed. If couples followed this policy, society as a whole would soon collapse under the sheer weight of numbers.

The answer to this issue is contraception. Contraceptive devices work by short-circuiting the reproductive process. In effect, they disconnect sex from procreation, allowing them to be separate activities. Thus, contraception makes it possible for us to enjoy sexual pleasure without producing unplanned, unwanted children. Effective contraceptive devices are one of the human race's greatest technological achievements, a significant victory in people's struggle to control their own lives.

ATTITUDES TOWARD CONTRACEPTION

Considering the benefits contraception has brought to humanity, the average man's attitude toward the use of birth control is unfortunate. Many men, particularly those who are unmarried, tend to think of contraception as solely a female concern. We assume that the prevention of conception is something we need not bother ourselves with, and our attitude toward the subject is characterized by aversion. This reaction is particularly evident when the birth control method in question is one for which we ourselves must be responsible. "Why wear a raincoat in the shower?" typifies many a man's response to the suggestion that he use a condom. The specious logic of this attitude breaks down under rational analysis, though: wearing a raincoat in the shower would be a very sensible precaution if the consequences of showering in the nude were as negative as an unwanted pregnancy.

Why are so many of us unwilling to assume responsibility for contraception? In part, the answer to this question relates to those exploitative masculine attitudes that formed the basis of the double standard. If sex was viewed as something men must get from women under false pretenses, then it follows that the male would see little need to take responsibility for the consequences of his actions. If women were the victims in sex, then let them be the victims of its aftermath as well—so went the basic rationalization for the lack of male concern with contraception. Sex is the man's business, contraception, children and the woman's domain.

True, few men are as blatantly insensitive as this. But the image of the exploitative, "macho," male has become, via popular culture, a sort of ideal many of us unthinkingly emulate. Thus, by trying to conform to what we perceived as a socially approved male stereotype, we have acted in ways that were a good deal more irrational and self-defeating than we realized.

The "macho" ideal left no room for us to feel concerned or responsible for conception and contraception. Instead, we had to concern ourselves with playing the part of the uncommitted, footloose seducer with little or no feeling of responsibility of his partner. This situation was likely to create a painful psychological bind, a conflict of loyalties. While normal human concern and simple common sense made us wonder whether we should be taking some precaution against an unwanted pregnancy, at the same time the socially approved masculine code would counsel us to "go ahead and damn the consequences." Asking the woman whether she was protected contraceptively was not part of the romantic, seductive scenario.

Distorted notions of human reproductive biology are another factor in some men's lack of concern with birth control. Because pregnancy occurs within the woman's body and not the man's, the responsibility for preventing conception is construed as lying entirely with the woman. In this view, the woman's becoming pregnant is seen as an inconvenient peculiarity of her physical makeup—an inherent weakness for which she has no right to expect special consideration. Pregnancy is a feminine worry. The logical flaw here is that while pregnancy may indeed be a condition exclusive to women, conception is certainly not. Intercourse occurs, or should occur, by mutual agreement between a man and woman. Conception occurs when a male sperm and a female egg, each containing exactly half the number of chromosomes needed to create a human life, merge and begin to grow into a fetus. Thus, it is clear that wherever the embryo may actually grow, the responsibility for triggering its development lies equally with the man and woman—as does the responsibility for preventing its conception.

Even if a woman tells you that it is all right to have intercourse without using contraception because it is not her time to conceive, you cannot feel that you are absolved of responsibility. There is a great deal of ignorance about ovulation among women, and since the majority of young women do not ovulate on a regular twenty-eight-day cycle, the most likely result of relying on an unsystematic use of the rhythm method is an unwanted pregnancy.

Another reason for the prevailing male attitude toward contraception stems from the erroneous connection some men make between virility and the ability to sire children. If a man believes that impregnating a woman is a way of demonstrating his masculinity, then he may secretly welcome the opportunity to do so. Actually, there is no correspondence at all between your sexual ability and your capacity to procreate, which depends chiefly on whether you have a normal sperm count and sperm motility, a factor that has no effect on either sex drive or sexual skill. A man may be a great lover and yet be sterile, or he can be quite fertile and still be unsuccessful in his sexual functioning and ability to satisfy his partner. By the way, many males prefer having a male child and blame the woman if they continue to have daughters. In truth, it is the male sperm that determines whether the baby will be male or female.

THE MYTH OF SPONTANEOUS ROMANTIC SEX

Some men avoid taking responsibility for contraception because they feel that to introduce such a realistic subject might destroy the romantic mood they are counting on to sweep away their potential partner's objections to intercourse. The woman is often guilty of complicity, for she too may wish to preserve the fiction that both of them are so carried away by sexual excitement they are unable to stop for something so mundane as a contraceptive device. Such self-deception is especially common in first intercourse situations, where excitement and anxiety are particularly pronounced. About two-thirds of the couples engaging in intercourse for the first time do not use any form of contraception.

The couples themselves may not perceive their lack of commonsense precaution as a result of their own guilt and confusion about sexuality, believing instead that they are acting according to romantic notions that sex is best when spontaneous and unplanned. There is no doubt that a sense of spontaneity adds to the enjoyment of sex. But spontaneity and planning are not mutually exclusive. And besides, an unwanted pregnancy is far too high a price to pay for the preservation of romantic illusions. But many are paying this price. Statistics indicate that approximately one out of three women engaging in premarital intercourse becomes pregnant. And one in four women is pregnant at time of marriage (for teenage marriages it is closer to two out of three). As a guideline, if a couple is not able to make a binding decision to use effective contraception, they are not ready to engage in sexual intercourse.

ACTING RESPONSIBLY

Once you have become convinced that you should assume your share of the responsibility for contraception, how do you go about putting that conviction into practice? Admittedly, it may not be easy for a man, particularly a single man, to actively concern himself with contraception. A couple's decision to have intercourse is most often expressed not in verbal terms but in a language of glances, signs, and body language. "One thing led to another, and we found ourselves in bed," expresses the experience of many couples. The problem is how to interrupt that nonverbal and highly enjoyable sequence of events with a consultation about birth control, and not destroy the mood that has been created.

There is no simple solution, but there are several things you can keep in mind that will make it easier for you to act. One fear you might have is that your partner will think less of you for bringing up a prosaic subject such as contraception while in the heat of passion, that by doing so you might cause her to see you as an overcautious, unromantic soul. It is unlikely that a woman would react in this way. After all, it is she who is in danger of becoming pregnant, so any precautions taken to prevent pregnancy are definitely in her interest. She is far more likely to take your concern as a sign that you are interested in her welfare. Thus, rather than eliciting her scorn, your interest in contraception is more likely to cause her to see you as a responsible and caring lover.

It is certainly true, though, that bringing up the subject of contraception can break the romantic mood. The point to remember is that the more naturally, unself-consciously, and frankly the subject is introduced, the less of an intrusion it will seem. Asking straightforwardly whether she is protected by the pill, an IUD, or a diaphragm is one approach. Assuming that both partners are consenting individuals who are aware of what they

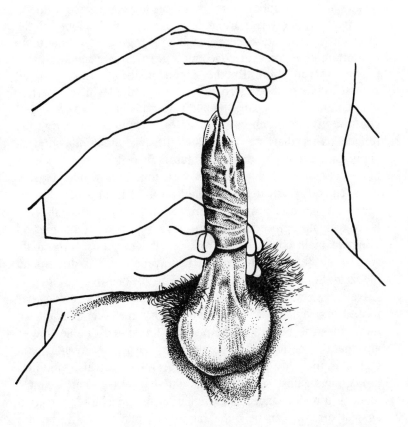

The woman putting on her partner's condom before intercourse.
Care is taken to allow about half-an-inch of space at the top
to accomodate ejaculated semen.

are doing, a note of realism, introduced in good faith, should not present an insurmountable obstacle for either the man or the woman.

MALE CONTRACEPTIVES

Another solution to this dilemma is for the man to provide the means of contraception himself. Of all the contraceptive methods available, only two are male oriented—the condom and the vasectomy. This situation results chiefly from the fact that more opportunities to prevent conception exist after ejaculation into the vagina than before. But the preponderance of female-centered contraceptive methods also reflects the attitude in our society that contraception is the female's responsibility. In the past, contraceptive research has focused on techniques involving the female rather than the male, and there is little indication of significant change in the near future. There has been talk of a new technique for a reversible vasectomy, in which a valve installed in the vas deferens could be used to turn the flow of sperm on and off; however, there are still many technical problems with this procedure. There have also been rumors of an effective male contraceptive pill, but it will probably be quite some time before such a product is available. It is difficult to block millions of sperm, easier to focus on one ovum.

Nevertheless, the male has no cause to feel that technology has passed him by, for the two contraceptive methods available to him happen to be two of the most effective and trouble-free of any that can be used. The condom has particular advantages in that it is the only method of contraception that also provides protection against sexually transmitted diseases. For a single man, or a man engaged in extramarital relationships, protection against disease can be quite important, particularly if he has several different sex partners. Condoms are available in most drugstores, where they can be purchased unobtrusively, and it is also possible to purchase them through the mail. Condoms do not require a doctor's visit or a prescription, and they are relatively inexpensive. The quality of condoms has improved markedly in recent years so that they now interfere much less with penile sensations. They are available in both rubber and natural membrane, lubricated and nonlubricated, and the newest varieties even come in different colors. Contrary to popular belief, very few condoms are defective (provided you do not buy bargain brands), so there is no need to test them by blowing air into them or by filling them with water. In fact, this is likely to cause damage. Finally, the condom is one of the few contraceptive methods that is entirely free of side effects.

To be effective, however, the condom must be used properly. It should not be put on until just before intercourse is to begin and the penis is erect. Some men make a habit of entering the woman without the condom in place, then withdrawing and placing it on their penis when they feel they are near ejaculation—an extremely dangerous technique that I strongly recommend against. Even if the man is quite sure of his ability to control his ejaculation, there is still considerable risk involved because well before ejaculation takes place there is a discharge from the Cowper's glands that contains enough live sperm to cause conception. This is why coitus interruptus is an unreliable contraceptive technique even if the male does withdraw before ejaculation.

The condom should be put on so that there is about a half-inch of space left at the tip of the penis to accommodate the ejaculated semen (some condoms are made with a receptacle end to provide for this need). Immediately after ejaculation, the penis should be withdrawn from the vagina, and while withdrawing you should hold the ring at the base of the condom to prevent spillage of the ejaculate into the vagina. Remember that condoms are made to be used only once; it's false economy to try to reuse them.

Vasectomy is a totally effective contraceptive technique, its major disadvantage being that it is essentially irreversible. Therefore, only a male who has had as many children as he wants (or as has decided he definitely wants no children) and has discussed the issue with his wife should consider having a vasectomy. (This topic is discussed in greater detail in chapter 9.)

MARRIED MEN AND CONTRACEPTION
We have been focusing primarily on the use of contraceptives among the unmarried. The rationale for this emphasis is that it

is among unmarried men that self-defeating attitudes and misconceptions regarding contraception are the most prevalent and pronounced. I assume that married men do not share these uncaring, irresponsible attitudes to the same extent as unmarried men, if only for the simple reason that they cannot afford to. Because a man is legally responsible for the children his wife bears, he must take an interest in contraception. Unfortunately, however, the attitudes and habits a man develops premaritally are often carried over into marriage. In no area is this more true than with contraception.

The majority of married couples have a difficult time reaching an understanding about family planning and deciding on an effective means of contraception. This is vividly demonstrated by statistics showing that one in four brides is pregnant at the time of marriage. Moreover, approximately 40 percent of children born to married couples are conceived without planning, and fewer than 5 percent of married men accompany their wives to the gynecologist for the purpose of discussing contraception. Research on marital adjustment indicates that it is best for a couple to wait at least two years after marriage before having their first child. Yet, the average couple has their first child after being married for only a year to a year and a half.

The main point that we, as men, need to recognize is that contraception is a mutual responsibility for the very simple reason that procreation and child rearing are mutual activities. To duck our share of the responsibility with the excuse that the woman's body happens to be the receptacle in which conception and pregnancy take place is both unrealistic and irrational. Couples need to be able to discuss their feelings about whether they want children, how many they want, and at what intervals they want them. "Letting nature take its course" may seem to be a more emotionally satisfying policy, but, as research has shown, there is no surer way to turn a marriage sour than for a couple to have children before they are ready for them or to have more children than they are able to care for emotionally, practically, and financially. After discussing their feelings about children, couples need to fully explore their thoughts and attitudes regarding the contraceptive methods available to them.

One thing both partners must realize is that there is no such thing as the "perfect" contraceptive. Each couple needs to be aware of the possible problems and side effects of the particular contraceptive technique it chooses.

TYPES OF FEMALE CONTRACEPTIVES

The birth control pill—the most popular contraceptive utilized by women—is also the most effective method of birth control available if the woman follows directions for its use and is careful not to miss taking the pill daily. The synthetic hormones in the pill prevent ovulation (the releasing of the egg by the ovary), and therefore pregnancy cannot occur. A woman taking the pill continues to have her regular menstrual period. It is crucial for a woman who is using the pill to undergo periodic examinations (usually every six months or once a year) by her gynecologist because for a minority of women the pill can have disturbing or serious side effects. For the majority of married and unmarried women the birth control pill will serve as a safe and effective means of contraception. It has the added advantage of separating sexual expression and contraception.

The intrauterine device (IUD)—which ranks second only to the pill in effectiveness—is a steel, polyethylene, or copper loop, coil, bow, or ring that is placed in the uterus by a physician. Once in position, it remains in the uterus until there is some reason for taking it out (for example, if the couple desire a pregnancy), or after two or three years in the case of the copper IUDs, at which time it must be removed by a physician. One of the advantages of the IUD is that it does not entail a daily routine, as does the pill, or application before each sexual encounter, as do the diaphragm and condom. The nylon strings should be checked monthly to make sure that the IUD has not been spontaneously expelled. Although no one is certain how the IUD prevents pregnancy, the most widely accepted theory is that it prevents implantation of the egg in the uterus. It should be noted that some women experience unpleasant side effects from the IUD such as irregular bleeding. The biggest dangers with the IUD are that it can perforate the uterine wall, cause infection, or be spontaneously expelled. The IUD has become a less popular contraceptive for these reasons, and if it is used the woman needs to be sure her gynecologist is expert at IUD insertion. At present, IUDs are more difficult to obtain because several manufacturers have removed them from the market because of legal suits.

A dome-shaped, thin rubber cup stretched over a flexible ring, the diaphragm is designed to cover the entrance to the cervix and is inserted into the vagina prior to intercourse. A spermicidal cream or jelly is placed in the rubber dome and around the rim of the diaphragm; the cream or jelly is toxic to sperm. When used properly, the diaphragm is a safe and highly effective contraceptive. It must be put in place not more than two hours before intercourse, and if you are going to have intercourse a second time, another application of jelly or cream must be used via a special insertion device. The woman must keep the diaphragm in place for at least six hours after intercourse.

The most common complaint about the diaphragm is that to some extent it affects spontaneity in sexual relations because it must be inserted shortly before intercourse takes place. The diaphragm has recently made a startling comeback in popularity because of its lack of side effects and because it allows the woman to take direct responsibility for her contraceptive care. Some couples make putting in the diaphragm a part of foreplay. Its major difficulty is motivation for use each time—many couples get lazy, or get swept away by the passion of the moment, or feel they can risk it "just this once." Also, women who are regularly orgasmic during intercourse, especially when using the woman-on-top position, are at greater risk for conception because the diaphragm can temporarily move away from the cervix. The practical failure rate of the diaphragm is much higher than its theoretical failure rate.

Other forms of female brith control include use of foams and use of a contraceptive sponge. Although these are somewhat effective, they are not recommended for regular use.

Since the three most popular and effective forms of female contraception all require a gynecological exam and a prescription, the next step, is to consult with a gynecologist. The man can accompany his partner to the gynecologist's office and share in a discussion of the issues involved. If this is not possible, then he could discuss her visit with her afterward and offer support for whatever contraceptive method has been decided upon. He should never delude himself into thinking that she alone is responsible for it.

Suppose, for example, that a couple has decided to use the pill. The man should accustom himself to the idea that, if his partner skips a day, it is not she who has forgotten to take her pill but rather they who have forgotten to take their pill. The same is true for the use of the IUD and diaphragm. Instead of the woman inserting the diaphragm by herself in private, the man could learn to insert it as part of their pleasuring activities. If she uses an IUD, he could make a habit of checking the string monthly to make sure it is in place. There are over twenty different types of pills and at least five different types of IUDs. While the major responsibility for advising the couple on what kind to use should fall on the gynecologist, the man can take an intelligent part in the discussion and decision. Working together as a couple on contraception can enhance feelings of mutuality in all aspects of a relationship as well.

The most extreme birth control method is abortion. It can hardly be said to be the ideal, since—religious and moral questions aside—it is expensive, is a minor surgical procedure, and can involve difficult psychological reactions. But it is sometimes the only viable alternative. When an unwanted pregnancy occurs, and the man and woman decide that abortion is the best solution, the man should support his partner through the experience both financially and emotionally. First-trimester abortions done on an outpatient basis at a clinic under local anesthetic are much to be preferred medically and psychologically. The same principles apply here as with other contraceptive techniques. The man must assume his share of the responsibility.

CONTRACEPTION AS AN ONGOING PROCESS

It is important to realize that the question of providing effective contraception is not settled forever after the initial visit to the gynecologist. A woman is fertile until menopause, which usually occurs between forty-five and fifty-five, and a man is fertile into his sixties and beyond. Therefore couples need to periodically discuss and reevaluate the contraceptive methods they are using in order to insure that those methods continue to suit their needs. Family planning and contraception are complex issues. There is good reason that they be seen as couple issues, where the male is involved as a committed, caring, and responsible partner.

6

MARRIAGE: CHOOSING THE INTIMATE BOND

Sadie Hawkins Day is a holiday celebrated by the citizens of Dogpatch, the backwoods community portrayed in Al Capp's comic strip, "Li'l Abner." During Sadie Hawkins Day, it is open season on males, and any woman who manages to run down, corner, and trap any unattached man has the right to claim him as her spouse. The holiday is enormously popular with the unmarried women of Dogpatch, who look forward to catching a husband, they would ordinarily be unable to obtain. But to the men, Sadie Hawkins Day is a time of pure terror, when each member of Dogpatch's bachelor population exercises to the utmost his talents of evasion in order to avoid what is generally referred to as "a fate worse'n death."

What makes the Sadie Hawkins Day pursuit so funny is its devastatingly accurate caricature of the male attitudes toward marriage in our society. Like the men of Dogpatch, we see ourselves as entering into marriage under protest. It is assumed that the rewards of marriage—closeness, intimacy, emotional security—are of interest chiefly to women. Men, on the other hand, value "freedom" and "good times." Women are supposedly involved in a continual effort to ensnare men into marriage, to deprive them of their freedom, and turn them into tame, obedient husbands. How close we are to the Sadie Hawkins Day mentality can be seen from the way we respond to news of a male friend's marital plans. The language we use in these situations is analogous to descriptions of defeat in battle. "Another good man gone," we might say, or "Another man bites the dust." Or we jokingly offer our condolences.

59

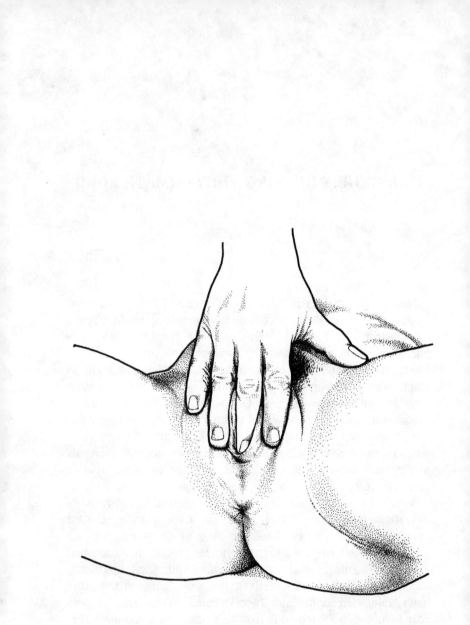

The man arousing the woman by clitoral sitmulation as an expression of sexual affection that need not automatically lead to intercourse.

The contrast between male and female attitudes toward marriage can be seen most clearly in the celebrations that precede the wedding ceremony. The bridal shower clearly looks forward to the married state. However, the male counterpart, the bachelor party, which features drunkenness and salaciousness in varying degrees, is a last look backward at the joys of single life.

THE REAL MALE ATTITUDE TOWARD MARRIAGE

But isn't there a discrepancy here? Statistics show that over 90 percent of the men in this country get married at some time in their lives. Marriage is neither going out of style nor is it a dying institution. Even with a greatly heightened divorce rate, it is men who enter into second marriages more often than women. If we are really engaged in a battle against the efforts of marriage-minded women to enslave us, then we must be extremely ineffectual warriors, since our losses are incredibly high. Either that or there is a good deal of hypocrisy in our attitude, and we do not really succumb to marriage as unwillingly as we pretend.

I think the second explanation is the more likely one. After all, it isn't only women who desire the companionship and emotional security that marriage is designed to provide. These are human needs, not just female ones. Marriage holds out the promise of a sexual and emotional bond with another person that will be deeper and more satisfying than is possible in any other relationship. Women respond to this promise wholeheartedly because they have learned from childhood to think of marriage as a desirable goal. Men, on the other hand, feel they must hold something back because marriage does not coincide with the image they learned to accept as an ideal. Thus, the average man may inwardly desire the rewards that marriage offers, but, for the sake of appearances, he must represent himself as simply another Sadie Hawkins Day casualty.

The trouble with this divided attitude is that a man who pretends to enter the married state under duress is apt to feel that merely consenting to marriage is all that should be required of him. It is typical of men in our society to feel that they need not put much emotional energy or commitment into marriage. For a woman, marriage is supposed to be everything, the very basis of

her life. For a man, marriage is merely one of several obligations, and not the most important one. Many men feel that
marriage is simply a matter of fulfilling certain set duties, and
that carrying out these duties adequately puts them above criticism. This attitude is typified by a cartoon in which a husband
and wife are seated in their living room amid all the accoutre-
ments of comfortable, middle-class married life. The man glances
over his newspaper with a look of consternation and says to the
woman: "Of course I love you—that's my job." Many men
expect and are satisfied with minimally involving marriages.

A marriage conducted in this spirit is bound to be unsatisfying. A man undertakes the responsibilities of marriage in the
same way he undertakes the responsibilities of his business, but
there the resemblance between the two institutions ends. A large
established company might be able to survive if the majority of
people working for it do their jobs in an uninspired, routine
way. American marriages do not have the extensive family and
community support available in cultures such as Ireland or
India. American marriages require a quality relationship to survive. There are no stockholders in a marriage, no federal subsi-
dies, no way of borrowing emotional capital. The marital bonds
of respect, trust, and intimacy must be built and reinforced by
the couple. Entropy, the tendency of a system to break down if
left to itself, takes effect very swiftly in marriage. Or to put it
another way, a love that isn't growing is dying. If the man is to
have a satisfying and secure marriage he has to invest more of
himself in it.

NEGATIVE REASONS TO MARRY

Because marriage demands such unequivocal participation, it is
foolish and self-defeating to enter into it with anything less than
readiness to work toward making it succeed. True, there is great
pressure to marry in our society. Beyond a certain age, unmarried
people are looked upon as being a bit strange, and single men
over thirty-five are suspected of being gay. Nevertheless, you
should resist social pressure and view marriage as one of a
number of options open to you (staying single, cohabitation,
group living, serial affairs, and so forth). You should choose to

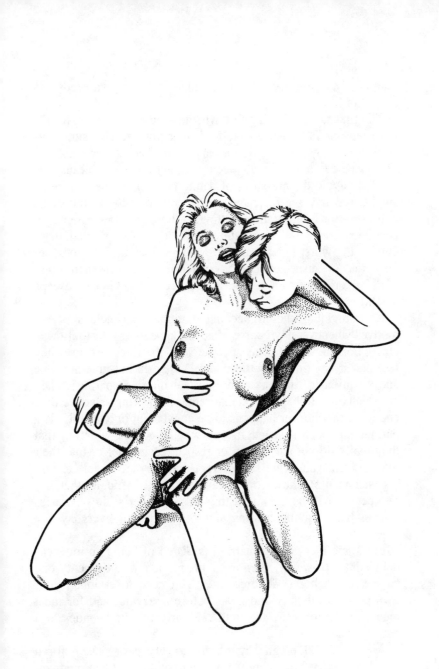

Another illustration of creative positions for sexual exploration
and mutual erotic pleasure.

marry only if you decide that marriage fits your own needs and values in life.

The first step in determining whether you are marrying for the right reasons is to ask yourself whether you are choosing marriage for its own sake or to escape from some other situation. For instance, a man may decide to get married because he wants to avoid the pressures of dating or the loneliness of being single. He may see marriage as the only way to get out of an unpleasant or boring family setting, or he may allow parental or peer pressure to influence him to give up his unmarried state. One of the worst reasons of all to marry is an attempt to cover up a real or suspected homosexual orientation. In such situations, marriage is not a positive choice but a kind of escape hatch.

An individual should become extremely suspicious of his motives whenever any course of action appears as "the only way out." For one thing, when people seek marriage because they feel that it is "time to settle down," they do not give the time and attention to finding an appropriate marriage partner. They are so anxious to be married that rather than being selective they end up with whoever happens to be convenient or available. If a partner has been selected in this way, a couple will find that they really do not care about or respect each other or that their interests and values are so different that they are unable to pull together in life. These strains can add to the difficulty that any two people will have in adjusting to each other's idiosyncrasies and in handling the hassles and confusions of everyday life together.

For some men, being married is a sign of being an independent adult. However, men who marry before age twenty-one have a much higher divorce rate. You need to establish your own personal identity and goals before marrying, and for most men waiting for marriage until the early or mid-twenties is a better decision.

An unplanned pregnancy is also a very poor reason for a couple to marry. Marrying the woman you have gotten pregnant may seem like the gallant thing to do, and such an action may have been laudable at a time when the price of giving birth to an illegitimate child was banishment from respectable society. Today it is a far greater kindness to consider marriage as a choice in and of itself, rather than as a way of avoiding having an abortion or giving up a child for adoption. On the other hand, it would be a mistake to go to the other extreme and automatically eliminate marriage as a solution to an unplanned pregnancy. The fact is that one out of four brides is pregnant at the time of marriage and that some of these couples make excellent marital adjustments—especially those who were already planning to marry and simply moved up the date because of the pregnancy.

Just as marrying the woman you've gotten pregnant is the gallant but unrealistic gesture from the male point of view, marrying a man to reform him is its equally foolish female counterpart. The woman who marries a man with a drinking or gambling problem or a man who can't hold a job, thinking that her good influence will cause him to reform, is being extremely unrealistic. It is the man's responsibility to change his life. Dealing with problems such as these is the job of therapy, not marriage. No matter how well intentioned a wife may be, it is unlikely that she will be able to reform the man. Nor is it her role to do so. A man who is motivated to change, and who assumes prime responsibility for change, can certainly benefit from a helpful, supportive spouse. But she can't do it for him; he has to change for himself with her help. One element of a good marriage is that it can bring out the best in each person.

POSITIVE REASONS TO MARRY AND CHOOSING A SPOUSE

So much for poor reasons for marriage. Are there any good ones? Yes, there are some very real benefits to be looked for in marriage, benefits it would be difficult to realize in any other situation. A good marriage provides a stable and emotionally satisfying way to live your life. Sharing as they do the high points as well as the everyday events of life, a married couple has an opportunity to develop emotional intimacy. Within marriage, an individual's need to feel loved, respected, and secure and to love and care for another person can be satisfied better than in any other human relationship. Of course, there is a dark side to marriage as well. Married couples can fall into the trap of boredom and psychological suffocation. The insights into one another's character that intimacy confers on a couple can be used to wound as well as to help. But when these negative effects occur, the cause can usually be traced to an insufficiently thought-out marriage decision, a lack of commitment to the marriage itself, or a lack of communication and continued sharing. The security and intimacy of a good marriage is one of the best experiences life can offer.

Just as there are positive and negative reasons for getting married, there are also effective and ineffective ways of choosing a mate. Perhaps the single most important element is respect—respect for the person and respect for the way you are with that person. With your marital partner, you will choose a life course—for example, what kind of family to have, where and how you live, the work you do and how it is integrated into the rest of life, your sense of life values. After the glow of romantic love has worn off (which lasts one or two years at the most), this bedrock of respect, trust, sense of emotional and sexual intimacy, and organization of yourself and your life are the key elements in a satisfying marriage.

A very important prerequisite to look for is the ability to communicate. Communication means a capacity and a willingness to share important aspects of your lives and personalities with one another, not just those that make you look good. A marriage partner should be someone with whom you can talk about your fears and angers as well as about your hopes and dreams. Letting your partner know about your vulnerable areas as well as your strengths is an effective way of building intimacy in a marriage. Revealing his weaknesses to his wife—especially feelings of uncertainty and inadequacy, or of sadness and depression—is one of the hardest things for a man to do. Males learn from an early age that they must always be, or appear to be, in control of the situation, and that women admire "the strong, silent type." Certainly, strength is an admirable quality in any human being, male or female. But no sensible person would expect a partner to be strong on all occasions. Your spouse must be willing and able to accept you as you are rather than as what she wants you to be. Especially important is for her to accept the difficulties and weaknesses you have without putting you down for them.

The involvement needs to be a reciprocal one. Your partner should not take the role of therapist or confessor. She should also be honest and open with you about her thoughts and feelings, both positive and negative. Effective exchange helps to locate the inevitable dissatisfactions and disagreements that occur in any marriage, and serves as a means of finding solutions to them. Partners should also be able to communicate happiness and satisfaction, since by doing so they can help one another to acknowledge the value and effectivness of their positive attributes and interactions.

Although it is true that after a few years of married life most couples grow sensitive to one another's moods and emotional states, they still can't be expected to be mind readers, and verbal communication remains extremely important. When joys and sorrows are not exchanged and are instead suppressed, the couple is neither able to fully share their pleasure nor to identify and work on problem areas. So, choosing a marital partner you can trust and talk to on both the level of feelings and that of problem solving is very important.

Another important guideline to selecting a partner is to choose someone whose interests and values are compatible with your own. If couples share interests, they will be more likely to spend more of their time enjoying life together. And while couples who have other interests work out agreements when differences of opinion arise, major conflicts over values that are basically unresolvable create strong strains in a relationship. Of course, your interests and values need not all coincide. It is an excellent idea to have some interests you do not share with your spouse. This gives you areas in which you can grow as an individual in your own unique direction. The strongest marriages are those in which there are both shared and separate areas of interest, where the partners have a lot in common, yet each brings something new to the marriage.

Before a couple marries, they should discuss realistically the major issues that will affect them. Some of the questions that need to be focused on are: Will there be children, and if so, when? How will the couple manage and spend its money, and what financial priorities will they have? Where will the couple live? What roles will each spouse take with regard to careers, housekeeping, and childrearing? How important is the role of sexuality in the marriage, and will the couple maintain fidelity or can certain types of extramarital affairs be tolerated? How committed is each patner to making this a stable and sharing marriage? What sort of contact will the couple have with their in-laws? These are core issues that need to be dealt with seriously before marriage, at least to the extent of laying down workable guidelines.

There is a strong tendency for a couple anticipating marriage to minimize difficulties facing them. This is especially true of younger couples, who feel that only by being romantic and by insisting that problems will somehow take care of themselves can they preserve the glow in their relationship. Building a marriage solely on romantic love is like building a home on sand—it will quickly be eroded. A marriage that is to succeed and last needs communication and planning of a highly realistic sort. Communication and planning are not incompatible with mature love, but are antithetical to the romantic-love myth.

THE PROCESS OF A SUCCESSFUL MARRIAGE

Functioning as a married person is, like other forms of behavior, something we learn to do. It helps the learning process if we have been exposed as a child or adolescent to good role models. It is beneficial to a marriage if one or both of the partners was raised by parents who were themselves happily married. For such persons, a good marriage relationship will seem the norm, and they will follow the patterns of behavior that were in evidence in their families. A person who has not had such good fortune, must adopt the opposite strategy and try to learn from the weaknesses of his or her parents. This person must work harder and more consciously to achieve a successful marriage.

Both Emily and I fit into the latter category. Our parents' marriages were very stressful and unhappy. We were strongly committed to having a less stressful marriage. We were so pleased with our initial success that we then allowed a certain degree of complacency to settle into our marriage. Both of us realized that we had reached a plateau, and that while we were reasonably satisfied, we were in danger of stagnating. At this point we made the conscious decision to work at developing our relationship further. This proved easier for Emily than for me. Like most men, I had a lower expectation of marriage than my wife. Trying to communicate more effectively, being more affectionate, and thinking as a couple rather than as a single person who just happened to be married took a good deal more conscious effort for me than it did for her. I have found that this effort has been very worthwhile, both for me as a man and for us as a couple. Several times since then we've gone through similar periods of reassessment, and I believe that these can be of immense value in any marriage. Marriage is like a garden; it needs a solid foundation, but it also needs to be consistently tended and replanted. You need to devote time and psychological energy to your marriage if it is to continue to flower.

Too many couples think about doing something to improve their marriages only when their relationships seem to be foundering—the "wait for a crisis" approach. If a marriage is thought of as an arrangement that is valued because of the emotional satisfaction and pleasure it gives, then it will seem worthwhile to try to make it even better, to increase the dividends it produces. It is a lot easier and much more fun to make a good marriage better than to try to lift a bad one off the rocks. Unfortunately, many couples do not try to change their marriages or go for counseling until serious problems have arisen and considerable anger, resentment, and a sense of hopelessness have accumulated. The old adage about an ounce of prevention being better than a pound of cure is especially true of marital relationships.

SEX IN AN ONGOING MARRIAGE

So far we have said nothing specifically about the role of sex in marriage. Obviously, it has a very important place, but only by first having viewed marriage in its larger context we can see clearly what that place is. One encounters different attitudes about the importance of sex in marriage. One viewpoint is that sex forms a sort of bedrock of the marital relationship—that if sex is good, everything else will be good. By the same token, it is assumed that if trouble appears in a relationship, the cause can always be traced to poor sex. Another viewpoint is that sex is of secondary importance, and that the primary element is the couple's loving feelings for one another. If their relationship is good in this respect, sex doesn't matter very much.

These extreme attitudes are simplistic and wrong. Sex serves a number of purposes in a marriage. Most important, it is a means of helping to create and reinforce feelings of intimacy between a couple. Sex also provides a form of affirmation and shared pleasure for you as both a person and a member of a couple. Also, sex can serve as a tension reducer, a refuge from the hassles of bills, children, and stresses of everyday life. However, sex is not by any means the sole and primary measure of a marital relationship. It is quite possible for a couple to have a good sexual relationship and yet have serious problems in other areas that can lead to the breakup of the marriage.

Sex is certainly not a secondary consideration in marriage. It is best seen as one aspect of a couple's pattern of interaction and feelings for one another. It is not something separate, but rather an integral part of the relationship. A favorite saying among therapists is that when sex is good it constitutes approximately 15 to 20 percent of the marriage, but when it's bad it can be up to 75 percent. Sex can energize a marriage or it can drain the marriage of positive feelings. Thus, it is possible for a couple to be intellectually and emotionally compatible and yet to have an unsatisfactory sex life, but it is not possible for them to remain in such a situation indefinitely, at least not without diminishing their relationship or putting it in jeopardy. If a couple is truly committed to making their marriage work and to getting as much joy and fulfillment from it as they can, they will not be satisfied with poor sexual relations, but will strive to improve that element of their lives.

A sense of closeness and intimacy is very important to a couple's sexual life. Feeling loved and loving is one of the chief factors that make a couple want to be sexual. Many men ignore this; they tend to feel that sex is a part of life that is completely unrelated to anything else. In fact, the closeness and affection two people feel outside the bedroom is of the greatest importance to their sexual life. For example, when a husband shows that he cares for his wife by expressing his hopes and fears to her, by sharing household tasks, by calling during the day just to say hello, or by planning a special evening out for them, he creates a feeling of closeness that will allow them to enjoy sexual experiences together more often. Intercourse is only one method of expressing affection and sharing sexual pleasure. In the larger context of marriage, sexuality itself is but one way in which partners express their intimacy with one another.

This point is especially important for men who feel that each act of physical affection must culminate in intercourse. Such an attitude, common to a surprising number of men, is an outgrowth of the tendency to compartmentalize sexual expression, to see it as a specific act that must be played out according to an unvarying performance script. When the expectation of intercourse is attached to every hug, kiss, and caress, the woman begins to avoid interacting physically, because she feels that if she's not prepared to go all the way, it would be best not to start something. Paradoxically, this attitude of "intercourse or nothing" is responsible for reducing the frequency with which a couple has sexual relations. When marriage partners do not feel free to express their affection both inside and outside the bedroom without the demand of intercourse, they lose out in all ways. The general level of affection and sensuality in their relationship is reduced, and they have intercourse less frequently. Touching both inside and outside the bedroom, with no expectation that all touching ends in intercourse, establishes a way of relating that promotes more affection, more sensuality, and more intercourse.

SEXUAL COMMUNICATION

Communication is another area in which the importance of a couple's daily interaction is clearly related to the sexual relationship. Partners who speak freely on a wide variety of subjects and who are able to relate negative feelings as well as positive ones are better prepared for the mutual communication and guidance that are necessary for good sexual functioning. Each person has the right and the responsibility to let the other know whether a particular type of stimulation is pleasurable or not. No matter how good a lover your partner may be, there is no way he or she can possibly know what turns you on unless you provide some sort of feedback. Men feel that they should know how to be good lovers and how to satisfy their wives without instruction or guidance. But, of course, the very theme of this book is that men *do* need to learn about their sexuality (and their spouses') in order to realize its potential. And both men and women have to put energy into communicating their sexual likes and dislikes before they are able to establish an enjoyable sexual relationship. Studies indicate that it takes couples at least six months to develop a functional and satisfying sexual style.

If you doubt that this is true, then try this test on yourself. See if you can name all the parts of your partner's body that she enjoys having stimulated (for example, breasts, lips, ears, shoulders, thighs, labia, clitoris). What sort of stimulation does she like in each of these areas (heavy, light, tickling, rubbing, kissing, licking, stroking)? What pleasuring scenarios are most arousing for her? Do you know her two favorite intercourse positions? What is her favorite manner of experiencing afterplay/ afterglow? If you feel unsure about any of the answers, then there are still things you have to learn, and the best way to learn them is by experimenting with different pleasuring activities and providing each other with feedback, either verbal or nonverbal. Men often feel embarrassed to initiate such exploration because they are afraid of doing something awkward and being rebuffed. However, this sort of exploratory activity not only increases your knowledge of each other's sexual responses, and thus makes you better sex partners, but it can also be an intimate and adventurous couple experience. It is something that can be done on occasion as your marriage progresses. People's sexual preferences change as they discover new areas of sensitivity and learn to experience their bodies in new ways. Couples need to communicate these changes to stay in touch sexually.

It cannot be emphasized too strongly that sexual communication in marriage must be a two-way street. Just as your commitment to the success of your marriage obligates you to be receptive to signals from your mate about what is enjoyable or not for her, so it is your responsibility to communicate your own preferences to her. To put it very simply: sex is a pleasurable activity, and pleasure means asking for what you want. Renunciation and self-sacrifice have little part in a sexual relationship. The first step, of course, is knowing what you want, and some exploration on your own as well as with your partner can help you discover this. The second step is making these preferences known to your spouse. This not only increases your chances of getting what you want but also diminishes your partner's uncertainty and anxiety as to how to please you. Showing your appreciation verbally and nonverbally can allay her feelings of awkwardness and make her feel good about herself for pleasing you, and she will be open to pleasuring you in the same way again.

It is important to distinguish between a request and a demand. A request takes your wife's feelings into account because it gives her the option of saying no. A demand does not. As important as it is for sexual partners to feel free to ask for the sort of stimulation they prefer, it is equally important that they not feel pressured into doing anything against their will. Sex is not good when it is coercive. Obviously, not all your spouse's likes and dislikes will be consistent with yours, and it will be necessary for each of you to make some concessions to the other. Imposing your wishes on your spouse allows you to get your way in the short run, but produces anxiety and anger in the long run. In these circumstances, the sexual experience degenerates into a struggle of wills. The negative power struggle that is unleashed usually extends beyond the bedroom. Even if one partner capitulates to the other's demands, the loser's resentment is likely to sour the winner's enjoyment of the experience. Remember, the object of sex is pleasure, not a struggle for power and control.

The importance of communication in sex can be seen most clearly in those cases where sexual relations between a couple stop entirely. The fault is rarely a lack of interest in sex, although one or both partners may pretend that it is. Nor is it usual that the couple find each other so personally unappealing that they have no wish to go to bed together. In some cases, they continue to remain on amiable terms in other areas of life. It is in the sexual realm that communication has come to an end.

Jerry And Fran
The suspension of sexual relations may continue indefinitely, creating an iciness that gradually pervades every aspect of the marriage. In other cases, communication may resume at some point, and when it does it is often with a bang, attesting to the intensity of the feelings that have been suppressed. One middle-years couple who came to me for sex therapy represented such a case. Jerry was an important businessman who was deeply

involved in his work. He and Fran had not had intercourse for thirteen years and had not touched affectionately for about eight. Fran wanted to get a divorce, but Jerry objected, claiming that it would damage his professional image and that he did enjoy the stability and companionship of marriage. Finally, both agreed to try sex therapy as an alternative.

During the first session, we talked about sexual communication and the value of nondemand sensuous touching. I described to them an exercise in nongenital pleasuring that I wanted them to start with. Neither seemed to be very happy about the idea, but they promised they would try.

When they appeared for the next session, I was surprised to see Jerry with a bandage over his right eye that did not completely cover a hideous, purple bruise. When I asked what had happened, they glanced sheepishly at one another, then, not without a degree of humor, began to tell me the story. Following my suggestions, they had begun their first pleasuring session by having a drink together, along with a few minutes of intimate talk. I had suggested they hold hands at this point, but when Jerry reached for Fran's hand she jerked it away, saying that they had not held hands for years and she thought it was stupid to start now. They hurriedly finished their drinks and went on to the next step, which was to take a shower together. Fran entered the shower first and began soaping herself. Then Jerry entered, and while reaching for the washcloth, inadvertently brushed against her bare shoulder. This triggered repressed hurt and anger in Fran, for impulsively she turned and rammed her knee into his groin, pushed him out of the shower, then grabbed his hair and smashed his head against the side of the tub.

Oddly, after Fran had gotten over her fury and begun to apologize for what she had done, and after Jerry recovered from his initial surprise and pain, their reaction was a shocked realization of how physically and sexually alienated they had been. They understood for the first time the strength of the emotions that had been bottled up inside them, and both felt strongly motivated to continue therapy and work out their sexual problems. Their ability to communicate improved so dramatically that they made rapid progress in therapy and went on to successfully revitalize their marital and sexual relationship.

SEX IN ONGOING MARRIAGES

Not every marriage is suffering from a communication problem as severe as Jerry and Fran's, but most marriages could profit from an attempt to make communication both in and out of the bedroom more sensitive and explicit. Communication, spontaneity, and a willingness to experiment are the key elements that can keep the sexual relations of a married couple from becoming boring and routine. Promoting these elements is the responsibility of both partners. Each has responsibility to communicate his or her own emotions, thoughts, feelings, and preferences, as well as to be receptive to those of the partner. Each can contribute to the variety and spontaneity of the relationship.

Where sex is concerned, this means refusing to fall into the rut of always using one sexual position. It means experimenting with different methods or styles of intercourse—serious, playful, quiet, excited, "quickie," or prolonged and romantic. It means experimenting with making love at different times of day as the opportunity presents itself, rather than adhering to the arbitrary dictum that the time for intercourse is just before sleep. It might mean having sex in other rooms of the house besides the bedroom—for example, on the living room sofa, on the rug, or in front of the fireplace. It means taking the trouble and forethought to add creative touches to lovemaking such as music, incense, lotions, candles, or an after sex bottle of chilled champagne. The point is that such variations and innovations are not extraneous trappings, but rather part of the act of love itself; they are integral in producing pleasure and expressing intimacy. They very much belong in the sex life of married couples.

CLOSING THOUGHTS

Ideally a man would marry because he wants to, not because he feels he should. He would enter marriage willingly and with his eyes open, not as the victim of some Sadie Hawkins Day type of pressure. He would need to have realistic expectations of marriage, not a romantic idealism or a cynical view that nothing changes once you are married. Every couple goes through negative experiences that need to be dealt with. A good marriage requires continued commitment, energy, and communication.

Once married, the man owes it to himself (and his spouse) to exert every effort to make his marriage succeed—not out of some consideration for marriage in the abstract, but because a good marriage can be a source of much pleasure, security, and intimacy. A successful marriage is well worth the thought, work, and energy needed to make it that way.

7

PREGNANCY AND CHILDBIRTH: IT'S YOUR BABY, TOO

A common cultural myth represents fathers as bumbling by-standers in the birth process, whose only real contribution is the sperm that starts things off. The myth has been expressed in countless novels, movies, and TV shows. The standard scene first shows the wife's coy announcement that she is pregnant and the husband's astonished response. Presumably, the decision to have a baby, the wife's missed period, and her visit to the doctor for a pregnancy test have all gone on without his knowledge. He has been kept in a state of strict gynecological ignorance, which continues to be his most outstanding characteristic as the pregnancy progresses. We see him fluttering with exaggerated concern each time his wife climbs a flight of stairs or lifts anything heavier than a quart of milk. When labor begins, we find him pacing the waiting room like a caged beast and pestering the nurse with idiotic questions. Presented with his newborn offspring, he is all thumbs and can scarcely be persuaded that the baby will not break if he holds it. If it is a boy, he demonstrates his readiness to undertake its education by bringing a football or a baseball bat to the hospital. If it is a girl, he does nothing, for it is assumed that as a father he has nothing to teach her. His only task will be to provide for her and to keep her away from predatory males.

Throughout the entire procreative process, then, the male is portrayed as not only peripheral but superfluous as well, allowed a place in the midst of things only because he is the one responsible for bringing home the paycheck that makes it all possible. The basic theme of this scenario is clear: women and

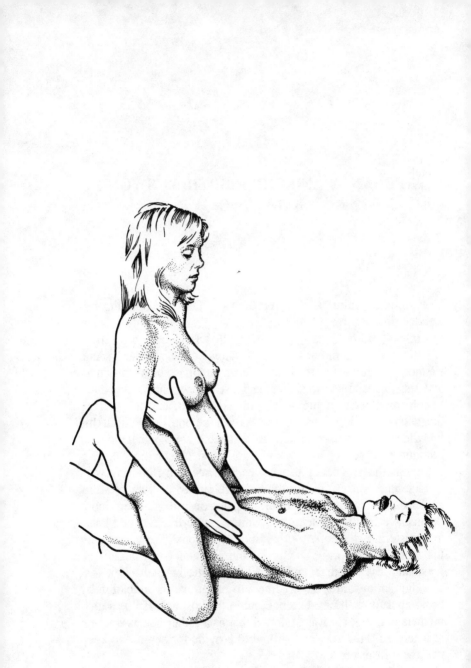

Intercourse during pregnancy. Except in rare cases, it is a myth to suppose that the fetus can be damaged by intercourse during pregnancy.

women alone are responsible for the bearing, and rearing of children; the male's presence is merely tolerated.

No man should allow his role as a father to be reduced to such paltry dimensions. Fatherhood is one of life's unparalleled experiences, and it can be replete with emotional rewards of a totally unique caliber. Because the experience is potentially such a rich and fulfilling one, it should be undergone deliberately, consciously, purposefully. Only by participating fully as a parent can a man assure himself of having taken the greatest advantage of the opportunity for emotional gratification that fatherhood offers. A man should choose fatherhood, savoring all that it has to offer, rather than just passively acquiescing in the experience.

CHOOSING NOT TO HAVE A CHILD

But choosing fatherhood implies that a man must have the option of choosing not to be a father. In the past, before the widespread use of effective contraception, before the population explosion, before the opening of the job market to women, it was taken for granted that soon after a couple married they would begin to have children. Today, however, there is no longer any reason to make such an assumption. For a couple marrying now, having children is increasingly an option, not an obligation. It is no longer valid or realistic to insist that the purpose of sex is procreation. Sex happens to be the way we conceive children, but it also serves other equally important functions: it is a means of experiencing pleasure, a method of reinforcing intimacy, and a tension reducer. Sex for pleasure is a normal, healthy, positive human activity. Couples should not feel guilty about enjoying sex for its own sake; nor should they feel that they have to have babies in order to justify their marriage, their sexual relations, or to please their parents and make them grandparents.

There are plenty of good reasons to decide not to have children. Having a child is a considerable expense. Hospital bills, visits to the doctor, baby furniture, and other paraphernalia entail sizable expenditures. As the child grows up the expenses get even larger. Clothing, schooling, toys, entertainment, medical and dental costs, and college tuition add up to an ever-increasing amount. Even if couples have enough to live comfortably, they should realize that the addition of a child will reduce the amount of money they are able to spend on themselves and thus lower their standard of living.

Some couples are unwilling to have a baby because it would mean that the wife might choose to give up her career (either temporarily or permanently) in order to stay home and take care of the child. Of course, an alternative could be for the wife to continue her career while the husband stayed home. In some cases such an arrangement might prove ideal, although it's still the exception. If neither the husband nor the wife is willing to give up working, hiring professional help to care for the child and the home, or using a baby-sitter, is becoming the trend for two-career families. But even with such assistance, the strain of raising a child while balancing two careers can be considerable, especially for couples in their twenties. The pressure often causes something to give way, usually either the marriage or the woman's career.

Couples who particularly relish the freedom and companionship they enjoy as a twosome might be unwilling to upset the balance of their lives by introducing a third member. Babies cut down enormously on the time and energy available for recreation. Couples who consider their social life and "fun" times indispensable should think seriously about the consequences before having a child.

Finally, some couples may decide not to have children simply because they don't particularly like children. Not being fond of children isn't something to be ashamed of. It doesn't imply that a person is unnatural or lacking in warmth. But if one doesn't like children or feel comfortable with them, it makes little sense to become a parent. Couples should also keep in mind that having a child represents a long-term commitment—for a period of at least eighteen years the parents are largely responsible for the child's welfare. A couple should take a long, sober look at this commitment and consider realistically all the obligations and limitations it involves before going ahead with the decision to have a child. Couples should also realize that there are several positive aspects of not having children, including greater freedom to travel, try out alternative life-styles, and live where they please rather than choosing neighborhoods because of schools and child-related activities. There is an increasing tendency for couples to weigh the advantages and disadvantages of child-bearing realistically and to choose childlessness if that is what they decide is best for them.

CHOOSING FATHERHOOD

If a man chooses fatherhood after thoroughly considering the question with his wife, his involvement in the childbearing process has only just begun. The major reason to choose to have a child is that it is one of life's special experiences. The husband and wife's decision is basically an emotional commitment to the process of childbearing. The next decision the couple must make is when to have a child, for ideally the arrival of children should be the result of planning rather than accident or chance. Potential parents must realize that the addition of a child to their family is no small event, but one that will place a great many demands on both the man and woman and will change their lives and their marriage considerably. Since the child will bring such great changes and demands, it is preferable that he or she be wanted, planned, and expected. If parents actively decide to have a child and are aware that its coming will involve considerable work and stress as well as joy and satisfaction, they will feel more positive about the child once it has arrived. This is especially true for the birth of a first child. Unfortunately, family planning is not as widely practiced as it should be. About four out of every ten children born today to married couples are not planned, and about one out of every four brides is pregnant at the time of marriage; for teenage brides, the proportion is two out of every three.

FERTILITY PROBLEMS

About 20 percent of all couples who decide to have a child will find that they have difficulty conceiving. If the couple has this problem, they should not feel embarrassed or abnormal. They should consult a fertility specialist (usually a gynecologist, endocrinologist, or urologist) to determine possible causes in *both* the man and the woman. There is a good deal of research being done in the area of infertility with new interventions to solve the problem. Couples need to be active and aware patients and work cooperatively with their physician. It is important that the man be clear about the difference between infertility and sexuality. Infertility means that the couple (the problem may be traced to the man, the woman, or both) is having difficulty conceiving a child. This has nothing to do with the man's sexual prowess, his identity as a male, or his ability to function as a lover. Fertility problems are stressful enough for a couple without adding to them inappropriate feelings of sexual failure. A man or woman who is bioligically unable to have a child is still as able as anyone to be a fully functioning sexual person. In my clinical work, I have been struck that infertility is one of the most stressful problems a married couple encounters. The process of doing the infertility workup (taking basal temperature, having intercourse on a rigid schedule, going for continual tests and appointments, surgical procedures, etc.) is time consuming and psychologically draining. Couples find their life is organized around the fertility problem, and each month is an emotional roller coaster of high hopes and bitter disappointment when the menstrual period starts. When the problem involves the man's low sperm count or poor sperm motility (the sperm are slow swimmers) this is particularly difficult on his self-esteem even though rationally he tells himself and the physician tells him that it is a medical problem, not a measure of masculinity. In about 40 percent of fertility problems, male factors are responsible. The varicocele operation is a standard intervention where the vein in the testicle is altered surgically to try to improve sperm motility. Medications and hormone pills are other possible medical interventions for male fertility problems.

Couples who are unable to conceive have to carefully consider the alternatives: (1) remain childless; (2) adopt; (3) attempt artificial insemination using husband or donor sperm; and (4) *in vitro* fertilization. In making their decision, thoughtful discussion between themselves and with the physician, family and close friends, and a professional counselor is advised.

TIMING OF CHILDREN
When should a couple have children? There can't be any hard-and-fast rule, but studies indicate that the most satisfactory adjustment tends to occur with those couples who wait at least two years after marriage before having their first child. It takes

at least this long for the couple to grow and develop into a close, strong unit. Waiting gives the couple time to work out a functional relationship based on intimate knowledge of one another's feelings, habits, and preferences. Thus, when the baby comes, they are better able to work through the demands that it makes on their life-style than they would have been if it had come earlier. A husband and wife who conceive a child either before or slightly after the date of their marriage have the task of learning about and adjusting to a third and extremely demanding person when they have hardly begun to adjust to each other.

UNPLANNED PREGNANCIES

Of course, when we speak of family planning we do so with some qualification. Nothing in life can or should go 100 percent according to plan, and this applies to the conception of a child as much as to anything else. Accidents do happen, even to people who use contraception regularly and conscientiously. When a wife becomes pregnant accidentally, a decision must be made about what to do. Should they carry through with the unplanned pregnancy, or should an abortion be performed? Husband and wife need to face this choice together. An argument could be made that since the woman carries the child within her body she should be the one to decide whether to carry the pregnancy to term. While it is true that it is the woman who must physically undergo the childbirth or the abortion, and while this may make her feelings about the matter stronger and more immediate than those of the man, it is still the husband and wife together who will be involved with the child as parents, and this must be taken into account.

Coming to a decision jointly can help to make the marriage closer and more meaningful for both partners. If the choice is for abortion, sharing it can also serve to lessen the burden of responsibility. Obviously, abortion is an extreme form of birth control, involving a minor surgical procedure for the woman and difficult psychological and emotional choices for both partners. It should not be chosen lightly. When an unplanned pregnancy occurs, the couple will naturally reconsider whether they want a child at this point in their lives, and, in fact, the majority of couples do decide that, once having conceived, they now want that child. But if it is clear that the arrival of a child (a first or additional one) would have a negative effect on the family, for whatever reason—financial, physical, relational, or psychological—and abortion may be the best possible alternative. "There's always room for one more" may not be a very good guide to follow in such situations because sometimes there simply isn't room. The fact that a couple is married does not necessarily obligate them to carry through with each pregnancy. Approximately three out of every ten abortions are, in fact, performed on married women. Couples choosing abortion might remind themselves that in the future, when conditions change, they can conceive a child that is planned and wanted. Or, if they decide that they definitely want no more children, they should seriously consider sterilization.

INVOLVEMENT WITH THE PREGNANCY

Once the decision to have a child is made and the wife becomes pregnant, several new issues arise. Should the husband be involved in the pregnancy or should he be the sort of ingenuous supernumerary we see in the sitcoms and soap operas? Well, when was the last time you enjoyed something you weren't involved in? Being a bystander isn't much fun, so why not involve yourself wholeheartedly in the birth of your child?

Pregnancy cannot be physically shared. It can, however, be shared in other ways. One way is very practical: the couple can make a joint project of learning about pregnancy and prenatal care. They can visit the wife's obstetrician together and take a prepared childbirth course. Prepared childbirth (also called natural childbirth and the Lamaze method) consists of a series of classes where exercises in which a woman learns to diminish and control the pain of labor and delivery are learned and practiced by the couple together. She is able to go through the birth process awake and conscious, without major anesthesia. The exercises are designed so that the husband will be able to help her in the labor and delivery rooms. The knowledge he derives from the course allows him to become a functioning member of the delivery team and, more important, an active supporter and coach for his wife.

Although only one in three couples now have children by prepared childbirth, it is a method that can add immeasurably to the emotional satisfaction of the experience. For the woman it means not only the chance to experience the extraordinary process of childbirth while fully conscious but also having a loving and trusted friend alongside her who has learned to anticipate and respond to the needs she has. For the man, it is something that helps him to feel a deep attachment to his family, a sense of belonging. This is something I have personally found to be true. Seeing my children born certainly represented peak experiences in my life.

CHANGES DURING PREGNANCY

No matter how deeply involved a man is in his wife's pregnancy, there is always that most basic aspect of the process that can never be shared—namely, carrying and giving birth to the child. This can lead to psychological and relational problems.

Pregnancy involves physical, hormonal, and emotional changes. While she is pregnant, a woman feels different from any way she has ever felt before. And this is something that may at times be difficult to share fully with a man, who never has had and never will have the same experience. As a result, a husband may feel left out. He can have the apparently childish, but very normal, feeling that his wife is not paying enough attention to him. This causes him to withdraw emotionally and sexually from her. These feelings are actually very common, and there is probably little that can be done to prevent them. What can be prevented, however, is the development of a major rift in the relationship because the man assumes that his wife understands what is bothering him and that she doesn't care.

A moment's reflection will tell you that just as you find it hard to understand what she is going through, she may find it equally hard to understand your feelings. The answer is to communicate your fears and hopes. It is your responsibility to share with your wife any doubts or negative feelings you are having, however silly or unmanly you think they are. Sharing negative as well as positive feelings is another way of expanding the experience of pregnancy and makng it more meaningful for both of you.

SEX DURING PREGNANCY

Pregnancy may at times cause the relationship between a husband and wife to become distant by interfering with their sex life. This is entirely unnecessary. Contrary to popular belief, a growing fetus is one of the most effectively protected things in nature, so sexual intercourse can continue without damage to it. In general, it is all right to have intercourse all through the pregnancy, including the last trimester, unless the woman experiences uterine bleeding, severe cramps, pain, or her water breaks. Except for those rare cases where the obstetrician imposes restrictions (for example, where the woman has a history of miscarriage), couples can have an active sex life during pregnancy. In fact, during the second trimester, increased pelvic vasocongestion in the woman might cause her to be more sexually responsive.

The type of intercourse positions you prefer will probably change as the pregnancy enters the third trimester. As the woman's belly gets larger, the male-on-top position becomes increasingly uncomfortable. An excellent substitute is the side rear entry intercourse position. One of the best positions during pregnancy is one in which the woman sits back (pillows supporting her lower back), with her buttocks resting at the edge of the couch, chair, or bed and her feet on the floor. The man then kneels between her legs. He puts pillows under his knees in order to bring his genitals to the same height as the woman's so that he can enter her comfortably. Once entry has been achieved, this is one of the most comfortable positions since it not only alleviates pressure on the woman's belly but also allows the partners to touch, caress, and speak easily during intercourse. Some couples find that during pregnancy they prefer a slower, more gentle style of intercourse than previously, and this position lends itself beautifully to such a need. Each couple should experiment in order to find the position and style of being sexual they are most comfortable with.

Childbirth is a strenuous process for a woman, and it causes severe soreness in the vaginal area. In most cases, an episiotomy (an incision to widen the vaginal opening) is performed, and this takes time to heal. Most physicians advise couples to refrain from intercourse for about four to six weeks after the woman has given birth. Not only might intercourse be painful during this period, but there is also a serious risk of infection. This embargo on sexual intercourse may sometimes be responsible for causing a husband and wife to become distant from one another. In fact, a first pregnancy (during either the three months before or the three months after childbirth) is the most common time for a husband to begin an extramarital affair.

It is the period immediately following birth—when intercourse is impossible and the woman is often very tired and is devoting most of her available energy to mothering the baby—that is the most trying of all. Rather than looking for sex outside his marriage, a more constructive course of action for a man would be to speak to his wife about his need for affection and for a sexual outlet. This is a time for both husband and wife to lean on and derive support from their relationship, not allow it to fade away. The husband who cares about preserving the quality of his marriage should consider altering his sex life during this period in a way that will not endanger the marital relationship. He could use masturbation to achieve the sexual release he desires or he could ask his wife to manually stimulate or fellate him. Under the circumstances, a man might imagine that his wife has enough to concern her and does not want to be bothered by his sexual needs, but in most cases this is not true. By expressing his desire to participate in sexual activity with his wife, a man can reassure her that she is important to him and that he continues to find her attractive.

Wendy and Phil

Wendy and Phil, a couple who had been seeing me for a sexual problem, found this out when Wendy became pregnant. Phil, an enlisted man in the army, was a rather nonverbal, unassertive fellow who found it difficult to request sexual stimulation from Wendy. After their child was born and they had to temporarily stop having intercourse, Phil found it hard to ask Wendy to manually stimulate him to orgasm. Finally he did, but his lack of self-assurance made him unpersuasive. "What's the difference between me doing it and you doing it?" was Wendy's reaction. Phil had to explain that it wasn't the same, that when she stimulated him he could look at her, touch her, feel close to her, and that this was very important to him. Phil's

statement was significant for Wendy in helping her to feel that
she was still attractive to him and that he wanted to be with her.
She felt she was "giving" to Phil and could enjoy his pleasure
rather than being asked to mechanically "do him by giving him
a hand job." There was also an increase in affectionate hugging, kissing, and caressing between them. As a result, their
weathering of the difficult first few weeks of the baby's arrival
was made easier.

FATHERING THE BABY

Once he has gotten through the joys and difficulties of pregnancy and childbirth, there is no reason why a man can't
continue to participate fully by learning to care for the child
along with his wife. Why stop at being an occasional helper
when you can be a fully involved partner in the experience of
child care? Such an attitude is, of course, contrary to the
traditional image of the American father. But in this case, as in
so many others, it is the traditional images that are cheating us
out of a great deal of the pleasure and emotional satisfaction that
are available in life. It is perfectly natural for a man to feel
warmth and affection toward a baby, particularly when it is his
own. Let's face it, like most young things, babies are adorable.
They are incredibly soft, they smell good (except when they
need changing), and they do amusing and endearing things. It is
a human response, not just a female one, to want to hold,
cuddle, and play with a child. There is no logical reason why
we should deny ourselves this pleasure just because of the
traditional notion that a "real man" does not show feelings of
love, warmth, and caring. A man can be nurturing and maintain
his sense of masculinity.

Learning to care for a child involves time and effort, but the
rewards gained by getting close to the child and feeling good
about yourself as a father more than make up for the work
involved. The best way to get involved is to make it clear to
your wife that you want to parcitipate and share the work of
child care with her. She can help you learn what you need to
know abut diapering, feeding, bathing, and so forth. If neither
of you knows very much about taking care of a baby, you could
read up on the subject or ask a knowledgeable friend or relative

for help or take a course in child care together. The active involvement of the husband and wife in raising and interacting with the child is one of the best ways of creating a truly intimate family life. A further benefit is that when the husband shoulders his share of the burden of child care the wife has more energy and attention left over to devote to their emotional and sexual relationship.

POSITIVE ADJUSTMENT TO A CHILD

Surveys have shown that the birth of a child is one of the most difficult periods in marriage. The work involved, along with the extra financial and emotional demands, can place a considerable strain on the marital relationship. In many cases a coolness, a sense of alienation, creeps into the marriage. Men frequently begin extramarital affairs, and in some cases the rifts that occur in the marital relationship eventually widen into divorce.

But none of this is necessary. The coming of a child is only a disaster when the couple is not ready for it. The best way they can prepare for its arrival is to go through all the necessary steps together—from decisions about family planning to taking turns at diapering and administering 2:00 A.M. feedings. Caring for a child is simply too much for one person to handle. In the past a woman might have received extensive help from her own mother and other female relatives. But since large, extended families rarely live under one roof anymore, such an arrangement is usually not possible. This change in family structure can be our gain. As men we now have a chance to participate in the wonder, excitement, and emotional thrill of birth. Guiding and sharing in the growth and development of another human being can be one of the most emotionally rewarding tasks in your entire life. It's not the sort of opportunity you want to let slip away from you.

8
SEX, YOUR CHILDREN, AND YOU

Obstetricians remark on the fact that a newborn male baby will, in most cases, get his first erection before the doctor even has time to tie off the umbilical cord. Sex is a natural physiological process from the day we are born to the day we die, and new research demonstrates that babies even have erections *in utero*. It doesn't take very long for babies to discover sexuality for themselves. Most children, both male and female, very quickly find that they can produce pleasurable sensations by touching their genitals.

During the child's early development, sexual sensations are not distinguished from other pleasurable feelings. Children become sexually aroused by experiences that are not specifically sexual (and so do adults—probably more often than we admit). An individual's sexual identity, feelings about his body, feelings about his genitals—components of his personality destined to play such a powerful and important role in later life—are in the process of formation during these early years. Children are not asexual, although this is still a common assumption with many people. Rather, they are learning to be sexual, and sexuality itself—the raw material—is there from the start.

PARENTS AS MODELS
A child learns to relate to his or her sexuality chiefly through example. The earliest and most formative examples are the parents themselves. Many of our sexual patterns, our sexual hang-ups, how we feel about our bodies, in fact, the beginning

90

of our personal and sexual identities is connected with learning experiences that occurred in childhood. This puts a great deal of responsibility on a parent. Most parents want the best for their children, and this includes a desire for them to have a healthy sexual adjustment. But we cannot help children gain this unless we ourselves develop a positive attitude toward our own sexuality.

OUR SEXUAL EDUCATION

Most males feel that their sex education was poor and generally negative. You need to be aware of these uncomfortable areas and be able to help your child deal with his own development better than you did as a child. The effort that we put into exploring and developing our sexual awareness and improving the sexual relationship between ourself and our partner pays off in two ways. First, we reap the benefits in terms of pleasure and emotional satisfaction. Second, we become good role models for our children, able to set them on the road toward the attainment of aware and self-accepting adult sexuality.

Few of us have had sex educations that come up to these standards. It is fairly safe to say that the majority of today's adults grew up in homes where nudity was prohibited, masturbation brought severe reprimands, and discussion about sex was confined to a brief, uncomfortable five- or ten-minute talk between father and son or mother and daughter in early adolescence. Often no real information was conveyed in this talk at all, just a vague admonition to "stay out of trouble." School sex education was usually absent or rudimentary at best, and the only religious sex education involved guilt and hearing no. Whatever information you received probably came from your peers, from sex magazines, pornographic movies and books, or from what you were able to puzzle out for yourself.

FATHER-CHILD RELATIONSHIP

As men, we have an added difficulty in achieving a healthy sexual identity—one that stems from the lack of warmth and communication between most boys and their fathers. Research indicates that both boys and girls report being much closer to their mothers than to their fathers. Women report feeling closer to their children as well as enjoying them more than men do. Generally, boys and their fathers interact only within certain strictly defined contexts such as sports or camping trips. One of the greatest needs of a young boy is to have a sense of what it is like to be a man. It is difficult for him to develop this sense unless he can talk with his father about his feelings, discuss questions about things such as changes in his body, masturbation, the meaning of erections, sexually transmitted diseases, and attitudes toward women.

A clear identity as a male child (which needs to be established by age two or three) will facilitate the boy's experimenting with traditionally "nonmasculine" activities such as playing house, taking care of babies, and cooking. If the father feels comfortable engaging in child-care activities as well as cooking and cleaning the house, this can provide an excellent and realistic model for the boy. As long as the boy has a strong identity as a male, he can have individual choice and flexibility regarding his activities and interests. He can feel equally masculine playing the violin as playing sports. A secure and solid acceptance of his maleness is the foundation upon which a boy can understand and adapt to his growing awareness of sexuality.

Girls, too, need a close relationship with their father in order to grow into a full and healthy sense of themselves as females. One of the saddest things in our culture is the separation between father and daughter that begins to widen as the daughter enters adolescence. She needs as much as ever to feel love, support, affection, and recognition of herself as a person from both her father and her mother. However, the father often avoids his daughter at this stage because he feels uncomfortable dealing with her as a young woman with her developing sexuality.

PARENTS AS SEX EDUCATORS

As fathers we have the responsibility of guiding and shaping the awakening sexuality of our children. It takes a special effort on our part to meet that responsibility, since we must first overcome the effects of our own inadequate sexual educations. Moreover, it is especially hard today because we live in a time of rapidly changing sexual mores. The puritanical equation of sex with sin and the age-old double standard are disappearing.

This in itself is a good thing, but it leaves parents in an uncomfortable and ambiguous position and makes it hard for them to provide guidelines that will be realistic and helpful to their children.

Parents have the feeling that they may be too liberal in one situation and too restrictive in another. Since it is a parent's job to set the limits of acceptable and unacceptable behavior for children, being able to tell what will have an effect on a child's development is particularly important. I will attempt to set forth some guidelines for making these decisions, with particular reference to the father. Some of these guidelines are based on research data and some have been developed through parenting my own children, all three of whom are presently adolescents. Of course, sexual attitudes and values will differ from family to family. It is possible, certainly, to be overly lax in setting guidelines about sexuality, just as it is to be overly restrictive. But between these two extremes there is a range of healthy and constructive parental attitudes and child-rearing guidelines. There are different ways to raise a child to be comfortable with his or her sexuality, and hopefully these guidelines will be helpful in that task.

FATHERS AND AFFECTION

Generally, men feel more inhibition about openly showing affection with their children than do women. Some fathers allow themselves to express affection with young infants, but beyond the kitchy-kitchy-koo stage, a father's hugs, kisses, and words of love become few and far between. It seems, in fact, that the typical father's ability to display affection diminishes in direct proportion to his children's growing consciousness of him as a person, almost as though he were afraid to be caught in the act. It is true that as a child grows older, he or she wants and needs less cuddling and holding. But a child (as well as the adolescent and young adult) never outgrows the need to feel that his parents love and care for him. If a parent ceases to express his love either physically or verbally, the child will have no real way of knowing that the love still exists.

Many children are aware that their fathers love them only because their mothers occasionally tell them so ("You know

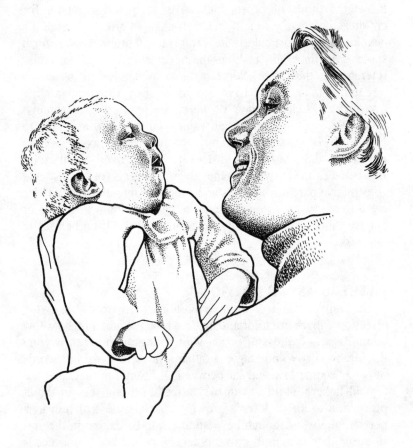

A typical expression of paternal affection. Unfortunately fathers tend not to continue such physical contact as the child becomes an adolescent.

your father loves you very much''), usually to counteract evidence to the contrary such as a spanking or being yelled at. This coldness on the father's part is justified as being an aspect of the traditional male role: it is the woman's place to be affectionate with the children, not the man's. His role is to be the disciplinarian and the task enforcer, to insure that they grow up to be competent, successful human beings. This lack of affection between a man and his children robs all of them of much of the enjoyment in the parent-child relationship. Moreover, it forces the child to live with the insecurity of never knowing for sure whether his father loves him, as well as creates coldness and distance between them.

But let's be fair to fathers. Most of us are not unaffectionate with our children because we are cold, unloving people. In most cases, mother is right when she assures the child of the father's love. Father does care. But he finds it difficult to show that he cares because of irrational fears he has about himself and his body. Let's look into the nature of these fears.

There is a common tendency among men to think of physical affection only in terms of sexual intercourse. Showing love through touching, kissing, hugging—in ways that are not intended to lead to sexual arousal and intercourse—is a form of expression that many men are relatively uncomfortable with. One of the most encouraging developments among young people today is the acceptance by young men of physical contact and even hugging of friends (male and female) as a sign of affection. But for the average man, unfortunately, physical contact with another human body is associated with only two contexts: sex and aggressive contact activities such as sports or fighting. The second of these contexts can be extended to include parent-child interactions, and perhaps this explains why the physical contact most fathers have with their children is in the form of roughhousing.

Sexual contact has no place in a parent-child relationship. In fact, there are very strong cultural taboos (not to mention legal ones) against inappropriate sexual touching between a parent and child. If every time a man expresses physical affection he associates it with sex, then he will naturally have problems being affectionate with his children. As there is growing awareness of the problem of child sexual abuse and incest, men have even a greater reason to avoid affectionate touching with their children.

Many men fear the possibility of becoming sexually aroused through physical contact with their children and so end up avoiding contact altogether. This association in the mind of the man between affection and sex manifests itself in different ways and in different situations, growing more and more inhibitory as the child matures. Many fathers stop being affectionate with their sons after the sons reach a certain age (as early as five or six) for fear that such behavior might be construed as being homosexual, or that it might influence their sons to become homosexual. Similarly, they stop showing affection with their daughters (usually before puberty) for fear of appearing to be lecherous, "dirty old men."

One of the father's greatest fears is getting an erection while playing with or being affectionate with his child. He believes this would indicate something perverse or unnatural about him. Although an erection is usually a sign of sexual arousal, it sometimes has no sexual connotation. An erection from a father-child interraction is not an indication that the father wants to have sexual contact with his child. It usually means he is experiencing physical pleasure that is not specifically sexual. Even if the man's worst fears come true and the child notices the erection and comments on it, it can be explained in just this way. There is no need to be embarrassed with the child or to feel that this is somehow shameful. In fact, responding in a natural, relaxed manner could be a way of conveying the lesson that the genitals are a normal part of the human body, and nothing to be ashamed of.

I want to make the point very clearly that I and other ethical sex educators and therapists are opposed to inappropriate sexual touching, exhibitionism, or voyeurism in a family. Most cases of child sex abuse and incest do not involve force or inter-course, but are a very negative experience for the child and interfere with healthy sexual development. Most cases of inap-propriate sexual touching in families involve brothers, cousins, uncles, and family friends rather than fathers. Although it is the girl who is the victim in most incidents, in perhaps as many as a third of incidents it is the male child who is the victim. Male children are less likely to reveal the sexual abuse because they feel particularly humiliated. There is a special stigma because it is a homosexual incident (95 percent of abuse of girls is perpetrated by males and 85 percent of abuse of boys is perpetrated by males).

There is a clear distinction between genuine and healthy affection between a father and his child and sexual abuse. Affection is freely given and received, is nongenital, is clothed, and is the genuine expression of warm feelings. Sexual abuse is coercive, for the man's sexual needs, involves inappropriate sexual viewing or touching, and creates uncomfortable and guilty feelings for the child.

HUSBAND-WIFE AFFECTION IN FRONT OF CHILDREN

Many men feel self-conscious about being affectionate with their wives while the children are around. Again, the stereotyped intercourse-directed view of physical affection is chiefly to blame. If a kiss or a hug is thought of as being a prelude to intercourse, then a man will feel strange about letting his children see him and his wife behaving affectionately with one another. If, however, he thinks of physical affection as a normal way of showing love and caring that need not lead to greater sexual involvement, then he will not suffer from such inhibitions. Thus, learning to be comfortable with giving and receiving affectionate contact outside of the bedroom can be very important, not only for ourselves but also for our children. Children need to see their parents being affectionate with each other as much as they need affection themselves. If affectionate behavior is a common occurrence between parents, the child learns that it is a normal part of life. These lessons will carry over into his own marital relationship when he becomes an adult.

There should be limitations, however, to the kind of affection couples display before their children. Certain writers have taken the extreme view that none of a couple's interactions, including intercourse, ought to be kept private from their children. But such a total lack of restriction on sexual expression does a child more harm than good. Children need to learn that a sexual relationship between adults is intimate and private. Teaching them that it is permissible to engage in erotic behavior when others are present is very poor preparation for later life. Sensual and/or sexual behavior between parents makes children uncomfortable. Many children whose parents pride themselves on being sexually liberated will tell you what a burden it is to have such a life-style imposed on them. With sex, just as with material luxuries, it is possible to go overboard in trying to give your kids the things you never had.

Instead of sharing their most intimate moments with their children, a couple would be much better off establishing rules of privacy that work both ways. In return for allowing their children a reasonable degree of privacy, parents can specify certain circumstances under which they are not to be disturbed.

Harold and Susan

One couple we know has three children—ages six, nine, and eleven—and has worked out a very satisfactory arrangement. After dinner, Harold and Susan often spend a few minutes over coffee having a quiet talk. During this time the children know that their parents are not to be disturbed, so they spend their time playing or doing homework, and if the telephone rings, they answer it and take messages.

A second aspect of the arrangement concerns the time that Harold and Susan spend in their bedroom. When the door is open, the children know that they may come in freely. When it is closed and locked, however, they know that their parents are not to be disturbed except for emergencies. The children, naturally, have expressed curiosity about what goes on behind the locked bedroom door, and Harold and Susan have dealt with this curiosity quite straightforwardly. They have told the children that while they love and enjoy being with them, they also need time together. When the bedroom door is locked, they may be just lying around or making love or simply sharing a moment alone away from the hustle and bustle. The children seem to understand and accept this, although they giggle and make comments. As Harold and Susan have found, if a husband and wife are going to be effective parents, they need occasional time away from their children. The most important bond in a family is the husband-wife bond; if that is attended to and reinforced it makes raising children much easier. It is good for children to be aware that their parents are individuals with their own interests as well as husband and wife who need time alone as a couple.

CHILDREN'S SEXUAL EXPLORATION

An important part of raising a sexually healthy child is for the parents to let the child explore, get to know and accept his or her own body. Parents need to feel comfortable about allowing the young child to touch his genitals rather than slapping the child's hands and telling him that what he is doing is bad or unclean. As the child grows older, perhaps by age three or four, the parents can teach him that while these self-stimulation and self-exploration activities are healthy and acceptable, they should be indulged in privately rather than in public. This can be done in a way that lets the child know that his body is good and that it is okay to touch it, but that there is an appropriate time and place to do so.

Many of us were raised with the notion that if a male child was allowed to touch his penis "excessively" there would be terrible consequences. Since no one could adequately define *excessive*, the tendency was to punish the child whenever he was seen touching himself for more than a few seconds. This approach can have negative effects, since if the child is punished or not allowed to explore his body, he can easily get the message that there is something bad or dirty about his body and/or his genitals. In later life he will have a harder time enjoying sensual and sexual feelings.

Not only is it normal for a child to touch and explore his or her body, but it is also natural for children to engage in sex play among themselves. "Playing doctor" or "playing house" are common activities for young children—expessions of normal curiosity and part of their learning to relate to other people. This body exploration will probably take place between children of the same sex as well as between children of the opposite sex, and also among siblings. It is not a sign of developing promiscuity, incest, or latent homosexuality.The time to be concerned is if the sexual activity becomes exploitative, aggressive, or involves significant (five years or more) age differences. Nonexploitative, explorative sex play is a way of learning about other people, both male and female. In terms of the parental role, a more helpful perspective would be to think of the learning that is taking place and how it will effect sexual development. Thus, when the parent overreacts and punishes the child for sexual exploration, the child is left with the message that exploratory sexual interaction with other people is bad or disgusting. A better approach would be to accept the activity and to interfere only when it appears to be forced or coercive or when it becomes the dominant form of play over a period of time. The parent should not stop sexual play by telling the children that it is bad, but rather by suggesting another form of activity. What this does is to give the child the message that sexual play is an acceptable form among children and that it need not be a source of anxiety to either the child or the parent. However, there is a time and place for it; not in public, not as a dominant activity, and not in an aggressive or exploitative manner.

PARENT-CHILD SEXUAL COMMUNICATION

Although it is traditional for information about sex to be conveyed through talks between father and son or mother and daughter, there is no reason why this same-sex rule should be rigidly adhered to. It makes a great deal of sense to have some discussions of sexuality as a family. This adds to the feeling that sex is a normal and good part of family life rather than something to be whispered about in private. Sex education can begin early in the child's life, growing out of his own exploration of his body, with the parent teaching him the proper names for his genitals. The young child can learn to be comfortable with words such as *penis* and *vulva*, rather than euphemisms such as *whatsit* or *down there* or *my thing*. As to the question of how much information about sex the child should be given, the best policy is to let the child's own curiosity guide you. This allows the child to pace himself in terms of what he wants to know or is ready to know. If you respond in a positive and open manner, the child gets the message that sex is something that is okay to think and talk about, and that he can feel free to ask again. Parents should not feel that because their five-year-old asks where babies come from, they have to tell him everything about sex from contraception to homosexuality. Try to give the child the information he is seeking at that time in words that will make sense to him. You establish yourself as an "askable parent," and the child can come back to you when he has further questions.

Perhaps the best form of sex education for children is a combination of formal teaching provided by school and religious groups combined with an informal approach coming from the parents. The parent might want to use one of the excellent books on sexuality that have been written for children. Instead of handing the book to the child, telling him to read it, and then asking if he has any questions, you might try an approach that allows the two of you to interact on a more personal level. First read the book on your own, then point out to your child some parts you found particularly interesting, or tell him about a misconception that you had as a child. Rather than just a question-and-answer period, the talk can be more of a sharing experience in which you impart not only information but also feelings, attitudes, values, and experiences. If this pattern is established early, it makes later discussions about sex more comfortable, as well as more frank and honest, especially important when you are in the difficult adolescent years. Discussions about sex can involve three-way conversations with both the mother and the father included. Family meetings including both female and male children can further increase the range of the discussion.

SEXUAL COMMUNICATION WITH ADOLESCENTS

Being the parent of an adolescent is quite different from being the parent of a young child. Adolescence is a difficult and stressful period when an individual makes the transition from child to adult. The physical and psychological changes that occur are rapid and profound. Within the space of a very few years, the child must adjust to facing a whole different set of needs, expectations, and responsibilities. Many societies, recognizing that this transition is both difficult and highly significant, mark the change with some sort of initiation ceremony or rite of passage. In our society, however, there is no single event that signals the transition from child to adult, and this lack of clarity about the status of the adolescent adds to the stress he experiences. As a parent, a man has a very definite role to play in attempting to ease the turmoil encountered by his adolescent son or daughter.

First, he must remember that an adolescent is in the process of becoming a self-directing and autonomous individual capable of making his or her own decisions. A parent cannot hope to exert the same control over the actions of an adolescent as he did when the child was younger. He can establish certain rules, set guidelines for behavior, but he cannot expect to always be aware of the adolescent's precise whereabouts or to supervise activities as he did in earlier years.

An adolescent must be trusted to make the right decisions on his own. One of the most important lessons that he must learn is that actions have consequences and that he and only he can be held accountable for the things he does. Thus, a parent should neither play the role of the tyrant, expecting to maintain iron control over his child's activities, nor should he feel overly responsible or guilty when his child makes mistakes. In either case, the parent would be performing a disservice to the adolescent by impeding his process of maturation.

At the same time, a parent must be aware that an adolescent is very much in need of support. An adolescent's first tentative entry into the world of adult freedom and responsibility may be exciting, but it is also quite confusing and frightening (for the adolescent as well as the parent). The adolescent needs to be aware of the parents' values and views about such things as dating relationships, petting, contraception, premarital intercourse, and sexually transmitted diseases. The parent should be aware that sexual behavior that is clearly inappropriate for a thirteen-year-old might be more acceptable for a seventeen-year-old. The parents must make a distinction for themselves (as well as the adolescent) about the kind of behavior they will tolerate, even if they do not support it, and the behavior they will not tolerate. For example, some parents will accept that their eighteen-year-old adolescent is having intercourse, but will not accept having this intercourse take place in their home.

Once these guidelines have been established, the adolescent needs assurance that both his parents—mother *and* father—will support and accept him. According to the traditional pattern, it is usually the mother the child can count on to be lenient and accepting and to comfort him when he gets into trouble, while the father plays the role of the stern disciplinarian. But there is no reason why a man should be any less supportive as a parent than a woman. An adolescent needs support from both parents, and there is no justification for a man's depriving his son or daughter of half of that support merely for the sake of fulfilling a socially dictated stereotype.

It seems odd that children, the living evidence of their parents' sexuality, should be raised in such a way that the knowledge of sexuality is kept from them for as long a time as possible. Sexuality is not something that is conferred on a person at maturity like a driver's license or the right to vote. It is with us from the time we are born and, like any of our other natural faculties, needs to be molded and developed through learning experiences. For you as a parent to deny this sexual learning process is to deny your child the benefit of having a parent as a positive model and to deny yourself the opportunity to be a sex educator for your children.

9
THE CASE FOR VASECTOMY

Although many methods of contraception are effective, there is no perfect contraceptive. We judge contraceptive devices according to several criteria: reliability, convenience, the extent to which they interfere with sexual pleasure, freedom from undesirable side effects, and, finally, the ease with which their effects are reversible. A method that scores high marks in a majority of these categories is surely worthy of our serious consideration. Let us, therefore, carefully examine the advantages of the permanent contraceptive method known as vasectomy, or male sterilization.

MISCONCEPTIONS

The idea of sterilization suffers, unfortunately, from some rather negative connotations. Sterilization has been used as a coercive measure to prevent individuals judged to be socially undesirable, such as criminals or mentally retarded people, from reproducing themselves. Hence, in the popular imagination, sterilization has come to be thought of as something that is basically punitive in nature.

The distaste with which some people view sterilization can be traced to a confusion between vasectomy and castration, a deeply ingrained fear in most males. Even though a man might understand intellectually that the two operations are totally different, he retains an emotional aversion for anything that bears even a superficial resemblance to the dreaded "loss of manhood." The fact that castration is used as a means of sterilizing pets and farm animals adds unpleasant emotional connotations. In thinking about sterilization, a man might be reminded of the family tom cat who was sent to the vet to be "altered" and thereafter became overweight, docile, and uninterested in sex. On the basis of these associations, he concludes that it is wisest to avoid any and all situations involving the close proximity of his testicles and a sharp instrument.

While such fears are quite natural and understandable, it must be stressed that vasectomy has nothing in common with castration, either in terms of the mechanics of the operation or in its aftereffects. Castration involves the removal of the testicles. Vasectomy, on the other hand, is a simple and safe minor surgical procedure in which the vas deferens, two small tubes leading from the testicles, are cut and tied so that sperm produced in the testicles does not proceed to the penis. The testicles still continue to produce sperm, but it is absorbed back into the body rather than becoming part of the ejaculate. The total volume and force of ejaculation does not diminish noticeably, even though it no longer contains sperm. Ninety-seven percent of the ejaculate is composed of semen, which is not affected by the vasectomy. The sensations accompanying ejaculation do not change at all, and there is no loss of pleasure. Nor is there a change in the male's ability to have erections.

Sex drive is regulated in part by testosterone, a hormone that is produced in the testicles and enters the body through the bloodstream. Testosterone production and distribution are completely unaffected by the sterilization process. Hence, it would be extremely unusual for a male who has had no desire or erection problem to develop one after a vasectomy since there is no direct or indirect physiological effect from a vasectomy. In those rare cases where a sexual problem develops, the cause is almost always psychological rather than physical. In fact, sexual desire often *increases* after vasectomy for both the man and the woman because their sexuality is no longer inhibited by the fear of pregnancy. To repeat, the only physical effect of a vasectomy is to eliminate the male's ability to have children; there is no physical basis for changes in desire, erection, or orgasm.

THE VASECTOMY PROCEDURE

There are some common misconceptions about vasectomy—that it is a lengthy and expensive procedure, that it requires a general anesthetic, that it requires a hospital stay, that it involves painful aftereffects, and that it requires time for convalescence. Actually, men undergoing vasectomies are amazed that an operation with such a profound effect on their lives can entail less pain and discomfort than a visit to the dentist. The vasectomy is, in fact, a minor surgical procedure that is performed in the doctor's office. The operation itself takes about fifteen minutes, and the total time spent in the office is usually less than an hour. The majority of vasectomy operations are performed by private urologists in their offices at a cost of $350 to $550, often covered by medical insurance. Many cities have developed outpatient vasectomy clinics where the operation is performed for a lower fee.

After administering a local anesthetic, the urologist makes two small incisions in the scrotum, cuts and ties the vas deferens, and the operation is over. The potential for side effects and postoperative complications is minimal. In approximately one in three hundred cases, a hematoma (blood clot) may develop on the testicle. When this does occur, the hematoma is either allowed to drain or is removed surgically, a low-risk, rather simple outpatient procedure. Present research indicates little evidence of any serious problems developing from vasectomies.

The vasectomy operation involves little or no subsequent discomfort or interruption in the patient's activities. There may be soreness lasting for one to three days after the surgery. During this time, the patient is advised to refrain from strenuous activity, and he may want to wear an athletic supporter. In any case, there should be no reason for him to miss more than one day of work, if even that. Usually there is a small swelling on each testicle, but this disappears in about a week and is no cause for concern.

USE OF CONTRACEPTION AFTER VASECTOMY

The man does not become sterile immediately after the vasectomy operation. Because the sperm remain lodged in the upper part of the vas, in the seminal vesicles, and in the ejaculatory ducts, from ten to sixteen ejaculations are required to "clean out" all the sperm from the semen. During this time, other means of contraception *must* be used to prevent pregnancy, and they should not be dispensed with until after the patient is checked by his physician to make sure his semen no longer contains sperm. For this test, the vasectomy patient can have intercourse using a condom, or masturbate, or have his partner stimulate him to orgasm and collect the ejaculate in a jar. He then brings the sample to the medical laboratory for analysis. A similar examination should be conducted again six months later to make sure that the vas has not accidently grown back together. This is an extremely rare occurrence, but the second test is an important precaution.

REVERSIBILITY

The question most often raised is the possibility of a "reversible vasectomy." There is a good deal of research and experimentation on methods to accomplish this, but at present a vasectomy should be considered an irreversible procedure. One technique that is being developed and tested is a spigot that could be implanted in the vas and used to start and stop the flow of sperm. However, along with the technical difficulties of perfecting the spigot, there is an added problem—when the sperm are not being used, there seems to be some decrease in sperm production and the viability of the sperm produced. Thus, even if the spigot were turned back on, the sperm might no longer be effective, and the male would be unable to impregnate a woman. If this technique could be perfected in the future, it would make the vasectomy the best birth control method ever devised.

With the advent of microsurgery, the success rate of restoring the vas deferens has increased. However, the structural restoration of the vas does not guarantee renewed fertility. So, although the reversibility chances are greater, if in doubt I suggest using another form of contraception. Vasectomy should be considered a permanent form of contraception.

One possible way of dealing with the irreversibility issue is for the male to deposit sperm in a sperm bank, where it is frozen and stored, prior to having a vasectomy. If the couple later decided to have more children, the husband's sperm could be used to inseminate the wife artificially. There is some question, however, as to how viable the sperm remain under such conditions, so that one cannot be altogether certain of success. Of course, another procedure would be to use donor sperm. This is a commonly used and accepted procedure in the treatment of infertility, but the husband and wife would be well advised to examine their feelings carefully before choosing this course.

ADVANTAGES

The irreversibility of the vasectomy procedure is, in fact, its only major drawback. According to the other criteria by which we judge the overall worth of contraceptive devices, vasectomy rates extremely high. It is almost 100 percent reliable, it is convenient, it does not diminish sexual pleasure, and it has no undesirable side effects.

For couples who have completed their childbearing, the husband's decision to have a vasectomy can be the beginning of a rejuvenation of their sexual relationship. Alan, a thirty-eight-year-old client of mine, married sixteen years and the father of three children, is a case in point. Two of Alan's children had been unplanned, and the problem of finding an adequate contraceptive method had been a major inhibiting factor in his sexual relationship. They had tried almost everything and were now using the rhythm method along with a spermicidal foam. Sex could not really be spontaneous under these conditions. Alan had never thought of having a vasectomy until a friend of his had one. At first he was reluctant even to discuss it because of his fears that the operation would make him less masculine or less sexual. Even though he realized that these fears were irrational, he could not dismiss them from his mind. His attitude improved when he read some literature about vasectomy and learned the facts about the operation from his general internist and from a consultation (to which his wife accompanied him) with the urologist. After much thought and several discussions with his wife, he decided that it would be the best contraceptive method for them to use. Alan felt anxious on the day of the operation, but found to his surprise that it was ''easier than having a tooth pulled.'' There were no complications, and Alan and his wife found themselves able to have sex spontaneously without worrying about pregnancy. Their intercourse frequency and enjoyment increased to a level they had not experienced since before the birth of their first child.

PERSONAL EXPERIENCE

Like Alan, the majority of men who have vasectomies find that the operation has a positive effect on their sexual relationships and on their lives in general. I know that this is true in my own case. One of the most difficult elements in my decision to have a vasectomy was the fact that I had been very much involved in Emily's two pregnancies and had thoroughly enjoyed the whole process of having children. A vasectomy meant giving up the possibility of becoming a parent again. However, we decided that two biological children and one adopted child were enough for us, and I went ahead with the operation. I have had no regrets whatsoever since then, and I find that being voluntarily sterile has given our sexual relationship a freedom it never quite had before.

As Emily and I did, a couple should frankly and maturely discuss the factors involved, and only when they are quite satisfied that vasectomy is the best answer to their contraceptive needs should the man have the operation.

CANDIDATES FOR VASECTOMY

Clearly, vasectomy is not for everyone. It would not be a wise choice for a young, unmarried man or for a man who is uncertain whether he and his wife want more children. Nor would it be the best choice for the man who is either divorced or contemplating divorce and who may wish to have children with a new wife in the future. But for a man who has decided, along with his wife, that he has as many children as he wants, and who wishes to be free of the possibility of causing an unwanted pregnancy, it may be the ideal alternative. Single, widowed, or divorced men who are certain that they wish to father no more children may also be excellent candidates for vasectomy. There are a number of men who see themselves as belonging to these categories. Each year, approximately 100,000 vasectomies are performed in the United States. Vasectomy is also gaining in popularity in other parts of the world.

The fact that vasectomy is a male-oriented contraceptive method, that it allows the man to take the initiative in birth control and family planning, is very much in its favor. Some men willfully ignore the fact that baby-making is a fifty-fifty enterprise and consider conception and contraception the exclusive responsibility of the woman. Male sterilization allows us to correct this distorted view by taking the responsibility on ourselves. In this way, we can make a major contribution toward establishing that atmosphere of trust and sharing which is essential to a good sexual relationship. When undertaken in a spirit of mature understanding and cooperation, a vasectomy can serve as a means by which a man lets his wife know how much he cares about her and is committed to their relationship and family planning. Of course, if there are serious problems in the marriage to begin with, it is unlikely that a vasectomy will resolve them. But if the relationship is already a good one, the husband's decision to have a vasectomy can and often does improve the marriage by providing greater trust and freedom.

DECIDING WHICH PARTNER SHOULD BE STERILIZED

The objection might be raised that the man should not necessarily be the one to undergo sterilization since such a procedure is also available for the woman. The two most common female sterilization techniques, tubal ligation and laparoscopy, are more involved surgical procedures compared with vasectomy. They entail more discomfort and greater risk. Although most female sterilization is now done on an outpatient basis with use of local anesthesia, it is still a more complex operation because it involves entering the woman's body. If based solely on medical factors, the vasectomy is the preferred operation because it is simpler and safer. However, there are more sterilization operations performed on women than on men.

Sterilization for either a man or a woman is best made as a joint decision. There are cases in which female sterilization would be the best alternative—if, for example, the man had a strong aversion to vasectomy, while the woman felt strongly committed to sterilization. A thorough discussion of the matter by the couple, as well as a consultation with a gynecologist, should precede any such action.

The same holds true for men. No man should allow himself to be pressured into having a vasectomy. If he feels ambivalent about undergoing the sterilization procedure, it would probably be best not to go ahead with it. It is important that his decision to have a vasectomy be based on his true feelings. The most undesirable consequence of a vasectomy would be for the man to be sorry afterward and to be left with a feeling of having been victimized.

VASECTOMY AS A POSITIVE CHOICE

The choice of a vasectomy should be made freely, with the man understanding the operation and its effects, and feeling comfortable with his sense of masculinity and sexuality both before and after the operation. Sterility is an unfortunate condition only for men who want to father children. When parenthood is not desired, sterility becomes a positive good because it confers upon a man a rare degree of freedom to express himself sexually in his marital relationship. Sterilization is now the primary choice of contraception for couples in their thirties.

10
NEW ROLES AND CHALLENGES: CHANGING
THE WAR BETWEEN THE SEXES

While presenting professional workshops in India, I began writing this chapter. India has a fascinating and diverse culture where most marriages are arranged and where males are dominant and females obedient. Traditionalists in India objected to many of the concepts presented in the workshops, saying the high American divorce rate proved that the double-standard approach to male-female relationships is the only one that works.

I don't believe the traditional double standard is either workable or preferable. However, it is true that the much-heralded women's movement has failed to deliver on the promise of "positive changes for women and men together." This is the time to rethink and redefine male-female relationships in a way that will enhance psychological and sexual well-being for both sexes.

So much of the discussion is and has always been ideological, moralistic, and/or highly emotional. Let us approach this most complex subject from a more objective, scientific point of view. There has been a great deal of scientific research during the past decade about male-female similarities and differences along a number of dimensions—physical strength, intellectual functioning, behavioral characteristics, health status, sexual response, and emotional and interpersonal traits. The objective research evidence is overwhelming—there are many more similarities than differences between men and women on all the dimensions, including sexual response. The same phases of desire, arousal, orgasm, and emotional satisfaction are experienced by both men and women. The same psychological processes of positive anticipation, the same physiological processes of arousal by vasocongestion and myotonia, the same rhythmic contractions of orgasm, and the same gradual resolution period occurs for both men and women. Of course, there are differences, but the similarities physically, psychologically, and emotionally outnumber the differences. The two major differences involve latency of response and variability of orgasm. The woman usually requires a longer period of time and more direct stimulation for sexual arousal than the man, although these differences decrease with age and experience. Secondly, male orgasmic response is more straightforward in comparison to female orgasmic response. The male will have one orgasm, which occurs during intercourse, while the woman might be nonorgasmic or singly orgasmic or multiply orgasmic, and this might occur in the foreplay/pleasuring period, or during intercourse, or in the afterplay/afterglow period. This does not mean female sexual response is either better or worse than that for the male, only more complex and variable. The crucial similarity is that both men and women are sexual people with the ability to give and receive sexual pleasure. Sexuality is a positive, integral part of both men and women.

TRADITIONAL MALE-FEMALE ROLES

Sexuality is an important component of masculinity and femininity, but not the dominant part. In the traditional double standard, men and women are given dramatically different roles with very little overlap. The man is socialized to play the strong, dominant role. He is the leader, the provider, the achievement-oriented person. The entire responsibility for the financial success of the family lies with him. He makes all the decisions outside the house. With children his role is disciplinarian. He prepares his boys for the rigors and competition of the adult, male world. For his daughters, his role is protector against predatory males who only want "one thing." His role is to make a good marriage for his daughter so that she will produce grandchildren and look after the father in his old age. In terms of leisure, the man has male friends he drinks with, plays cards with, and watches sports with. The man depends on the woman to take care of his food, clothes, and health needs.

In the stereotypic double standard socialization, the woman takes the role of the weaker, dependent spouse. Her role is to nurture and take care of her husband and children, and she is expected to derive her self-esteem from their accomplishments. Her domain is the home—organizing, cooking, and cleaning. Most important, she is responsible for her family's emotional needs; she is the prime (and usually only) caretaker. Sexual pleasure is his domain, not hers, but if she is to experience arousal it has to occur during intercourse. If she has an orgasm it has to be just like the man's—a single orgasm during intercourse. If she is to work outside the home, it is only for extra money for the family, not to pursue her own career. She is not expected to have intellectual interests. Her only friends are other women and relatives. She is in charge of the couple's social life with other couples and families, but is not to have male friends because such relationships would undoubtedly turn into extramarital affairs (after all, why would a man want to have a friendship with a woman other than to have a sexual affair with her?).

These rigid stereotyped male-female roles had a negative effect on the couple's emotional and sexual relationship, but just as important, they inhibited the personal growth of the man and the woman. Everyone, including children, loses out in relationships based on these rigid, irrational roles.

It is always easier to tear down an old system than to develop a new model that is more rational, functional, and satisfying. I am not suggesting that the model I'm presenting is perfect, or the only one, or that it will work for all males or all couples. What will be proposed is a model of male-female relationships that is congruent with scientific information about the similarities between men and women and that has demonstrated positive potential to enhance emotional and sexual satisfaction.

A NEW MODEL OF MALE-FEMALE RELATIONSHIPS

The foundation is a respectful view of the female as being a competent and sexual person. The model is not one of fifty-fifty equality in every aspect of life (which is overly idealistic and doomed to failure). Rather, it is based on a sense of equity between men and women. One person might have prime responsibility or skill in one area and the other might have prime responsibility and skill in another area. The prime element is that the man and woman relate to each other as respectful human beings who value each other's competence and share power in an equitable manner. When they relate as respectful, equitable, and caring partners it serves as an excellent model for children to learn about male-female relationships. People who treat each other well outside the bedroom will usually treat each other well inside the bedroom also.

The second dimension revolves around trust between men and women. Instead of men and women being at war, seeing the opposite sex as the enemy trying to dominate you, in this relationship you trust that the woman will not do something to purposely undercut or harm you. You view her as having your best interests in mind and as your friend and supporter. For trust to be genuine, it must be reciprocal. The woman needs to have that same degree of trust in your motivations and behavior. Trust does not mean that at times there will not be problems, disappointments, and anger. It does mean you relate to one another in a trusting way, not doing something to intentionally hurt your partner, but trying to act in her best interest.

The third building block is a sense of caring and intimacy between the man and woman. This is a more solid and more mature basis for a relationship than the romantic love phenomenon glorified in movies and books. Romantic love is passionate and all-consuming. It offers the promise of bliss, "never having to say you're sorry," and it usually ends in a bitter, destructive manner. It makes great fiction, but is a very hard and unsuitable way to conduct your life. Our new model of intimacy sees the choice of a romantic relationship as based partly in emotion, but more firmly in a realistic view of the woman (in terms of respect, trust, and communicating about a range of issues) and a belief that you as a couple can plan and develop a joint life together. Your caring for each other would be deep as well as passionate. Intimacy would be more than sexual and would include sharing thoughts, feelings, beliefs, values, and plans. Sexuality between a man and a woman is an integral part of a relationship. Sex serves to energize a relationship by reinforcing and deepening intimacy. Contrary to traditional male beliefs, sex is not the most important thing in a relationship but partners need to view each other as sexual people and participate in sex in a respectful, trusting, caring, and cooperative way.

The ability to listen and respond empathically to each other's thoughts and feelings is important. Being able to clearly and directly state your feelings and make requests (not demands) of your partner is vital. It is crucial to deal with problems rather than avoid them, and to use good problem-solving skills (clearly stating your feelings about the problem, developing alternatives, objectively evaluating the pros and cons of each, committing yourself to a solution, implementing the solution, and monitoring the results) and act in a constructive, goal-oriented manner. In addition, a relationship between a man and a woman includes toleration and humor to get past the difficult situations and hard times.

The most intimate and involving relationship between a man and a woman is marriage, where these skills and attitudes play their most crucial role. However, elements of our model of male-female relationships are relevant to work, friendships, family, and other social situations.

Tom and Nancy

Tom and Nancy, a married couple for eighteen years, with a fourteen-year-old daughter, provide a good example of this new model of male-female relationships in practice. Tom came from a working-class family characterized by a great deal of violence, including spouse and child abuse. When Tom was seven his father died in a car accident, driving while intoxicated. His mother moved the children to the medium-size city where her parents lived. Tom grew up around uncles and his grandfather, but did not have a positive male model.

A turning point occurred in Tom's life when he was a seventeen-year-old high school junior. A freshman girl who was very immature and desperately wanted attention would go with boys into the woods and engage in oral sex (giving "blow jobs"). One day, Tom was with three of his friends who were joking and bragging about how this was "what life really had to offer." Tom, like most of the boys in his town, had been to a prostitute a couple of times. In his social group being a virgin after sixteen was ridiculed, and you had to prove you weren't a "fag." However, in viewing the scene with the freshman girl, Tom knew it was not for him. Although he wasn't assertive enough at that time in his life to say anything (a fact he regrets when looking back on the incident), he did choose not to get involved in the kind of sexual activity where a woman is used and abused.

Tom talked to his favorite female teacher about that incident and about his future plans. Good teachers earn their pay not just in the classroom but in listening to and guiding adolescents outside the classroom. She encouraged Tom to use his intellectual ability to advance himself by getting a college education. She also explained to him that one of the major reasons students in the town did not go on for further schooling or training was unwanted, unplanned pregnancies that resulted in early marriages. She suggested that at a minimum he use condoms. For the first time, Tom was introduced to the idea that women were sexual people, not sex objects, and that a dating relationship should be based on the concept of a respectful friendship with the adolescent female. You trust a friend will like you and not do anything to hurt you—shouldn't this also apply to a male-female dating and sexual relationship?

Although Tom continued to kid around with his old male friends, he started choosing new male and female friends who took a more serious and responsible view toward life. After he graduated high school, he attended the local community college for two years and eventually graduated from the state university. College had a good effect on Tom. He majored in personnel management, and worked during the summers as a clerk in a personnel department. Tom became aware of the feelings engendered by being treated as a "second-class citizen" and saw that often even professional women were treated that way.

Tom resolved not to marry until he was established in his career, which he believed meant at least age thirty. He enjoyed a moderately active dating and sexual life, typically dating one person at a time. The affairs usually lasted from six months to two years. Before beginning intercourse, he always made sure the woman was using birth control pills, or had an IUD, or used her diaphragm. If not, he would always use a condom. Although he had two relationships that ended bitterly, most were good ones where he felt he had been a respectful friend with the woman and that he'd learned about himself.

After college, he received an assistantship to study for a master's degree in industrial relations. One of the women in his graduate program was Nancy. At first they related as professional friends, both because Nancy was involved in a romance and because Tom was a bit intimidated by Nancy's academic excellence. However, Tom did invite her to dinner after the semester ended, and they talked long into the night about personal and professional plans. Tom was aware of his sexual attraction to Nancy and put in the back of his head that he would like to date her if there was ever an opportunity. During the next semester, they saw each other two or three times a week as platonic friends discussing academic subjects. Toward the end of the semester they joined a coed volleyball team with a group of other students. Nancy met the woman Tom was dating and he met the man Nancy was involved with. Tom wondered to himself what attracted Nancy to this fellow, since he drank too much and treated her badly. As she confided to Tom: "He treats me like shit and I don't know why I put up with it." Tom didn't, either, but it took her off the pedestal Tom had put her on.

Dinner after semester exams was becoming a tradition with Tom and Nancy, and after drinking too much wine (not a recommended behavior to initiate self-disclosure, but a pretty common one for males), Tom told Nancy the story of his father's death and his teacher's advice. Nancy was a very concerned listener, and this emboldened Tom to tell her how attracted he felt toward her. Nancy was receptive, and the evening was a romantic, sensuous one—but one that did not culminate in intercourse. The next day Tom called and invited her for a walk in the park. Tom told her that his feelings of the previous night were genuine, that it was not the wine talking. However, if they were to become a romantic couple Tom wanted Nancy to first make a clean break from her current lover. He didn't want a messy scene where he would try to take her away and she would vacillate back and forth. Nancy was angry at Tom because she was hoping a new relationship would give her the impetus to get out of the self-defeating one. However, she realized Tom was right, it was her responsibility to break off the old affair, and that she should not use Tom as an excuse. It took Nancy a full six weeks to do it, and during that time Tom continued to support but not force her.

Once they began as a romantic and sexual couple, it was passionate and fun. They did all the special things lovers do— stay up for hours talking, spend the next day in bed making love, eat popcorn for breakfast, make love at midnight on the beach, and dream of the perfect marriage and life. Romantic love is an experience not to be missed, but at best it only lasts a year or two. Romantic love is not a basis for marriage.

After graduation, Tom and Nancy did two very hard but necessary things. They visited each other's families and talked frankly about the elements in their backgrounds they admired and wanted to have in their own marriage and family, and the elements that were "traps" for them (i.e., things they would have to be careful to avoid). For Tom, the trap was playing the dominant role and looking at the woman as "weak, pure, and having to be taken care of." Nancy came from an alcoholic family where her stepbrother had sexually abused her between ages eleven and thirteen. She had a hard time trusting men, and although she was self-confident academically, her personal and sexual self-esteem was too dependent on the approval of others. One aspect of a good relationship is that it brings out the best in each person. Nancy wanted Tom to see himself as a competent man, but also as someone who could work with others in a respectful, cooperative manner rather than dominate them. Tom wanted Nancy to see herself as a survivor, not a victim. She needed to trust herself and trust him, and build personal and sexual self-esteem.

The second hard thing was to decide about career issues and where to live. The old system in which the man's career always came first might not promote male-female equity, but it was certainly easier. It is hard to coordinate two careers, especially when both people are in the same field. Tom and Nancy agreed to look at all alternatives and make decisions that took into account both their needs. They were not so naive to believe all decisions would be equal or that making them would be easy. They chose to look for jobs in the three large cities that they both would have liked to live in. Each had a veto power—although Tom would have liked New York, Nancy found it too expensive and hectic. Nancy liked the idea of Dallas or Houston, but Tom wanted to avoid Texas for work-related reasons. They settled on Washington, D.C. This concept of each having a veto power over important life decisions has served them well. For instance, six years into their marriage, Tom was interested in having a second child, but Nancy vetoed the idea since she felt that with their careers, activities, and marriage a second child would decrease the quality of their life and family. A hard decision, but having a child entails a strong, mutual commitment from both partners. Tom realized he could not force Nancy to have a second child.

In deciding to marry, they made a strong commitment to making the marriage work, but agreed they would not stay together for tradition, or dependency, or for the sake of a child if the marriage was a destructive one. This agreement served to maintain their commitment toward making their marital bond a respectful, trusting, and intimate one. They would not take the marriage for granted and allow it to stagnate. Sexuality plays an integral role in energizing their marriage and maintaining a sense of intimate emotional contact.

A marriage (and marital sex) needs consistent attention and a sense of growth and development. Nancy and Tom need to change and grow as individual people and their marriage needs to be both cohesive and flexible to adjust to these personal changes. For an emotional and sexual relationship to thrive, both people have to be good listeners, be clear and direct in stating their opinions and making requests, look at a range of alternatives when facing a problem, and make decisions in a respectful manner so they reach an agreement both can live with. The latter has been particularly crucial in terms of balancing career issues and raising their child. Tom would have preferred Nancy to have been a more traditional, less ambitious professional person. However, he had to admit that her influence and questioning made him a more aware and involved professional, unlike many of his colleagues who appeared "burned-out" in their jobs by age forty. The security of a second income allowed Tom to take professional risks (i.e., setting up his own consulting firm, which he might not have done if he were the primary or sole provider). On the other hand, he regretted not having the flexibility to change locations for a better job opportunity. Life is a series of problem-solving opportunities where you make the best decisions based on realistic alternatives, not an ideal world where you have total control and can have it all.

Tom was more involved in the nitty-gritty tasks of child raising than he ever imagined he would be. From changing diapers, to going to school open houses, to taking his daughter shopping, to talking to her about friendships with both boys and girls, Tom was an involved parent. He found parts of it aggravating, such as driving car pools and waiting around, but other parts tremendously gratifying, such as helping her prepare for her first dance (since Nancy was out of town on business). Tom felt sorry for his male friends who were only marginally involved in parenting.

As Tom and Nancy look toward their future, they're aware that life will continue to present them with challenges and change. They spend time talking, planning, and developing goals for the second part of their lives. They look forward to launching their daughter into college and adulthood and have no fear of the "empty nest" syndrome. They plan to pursue individual interests—Tom to write a book advocating changing policies concerning maternity/paternity leave and flexible work hours and Nancy to run for the city council. Tom hopes to pursue his interest in hiking (which Nancy shares with him) and his hobby of golf, while Nancy pursues her interest in quilting. As a couple they plan to travel and do social justice projects with their church group.

GUIDELINES FOR MALE-FEMALE RELATIONSHIPS

Tom and Nancy are not the perfect couple, but they have achieved much that is admirable. In part that comes from following basic guidelines about male-female relationships that can be enhancing for both sexes:

1. A respectful attitude toward women that sees them as equal people.
2. An open and flexible attitude toward male-female roles.
3. An acceptance and security about yourself and your mas-

culinity so you are not threatened or intimidated by women.

4. A realization that intellectually, emotionally, and sexually there are more similarities than differences between men and women.

5. An ability to see that you can have a professional and/or personal friendship with a woman; do not sexualize all male-female relationships.

6. A feeling that you can be comfortable and confident in your masculinity, so that some of the activities or interests that have traditionally been labeled "feminine" can be integrated into your life.

7. A realization that a intimate sexual relationship will be more satisfying if both of you can initiate and enjoy the whole range of sexual pleasures.

8. An attitude that conception, contraception, and children are as much the domain of the man as the woman.

9. Knowledge that a respectful, equitable, trusting, and intimate marriage is the most satisfying kind.

10. Recognition that a communicative, sharing, and giving relationship between a man and a woman promotes emotional and sexual satisfaction.

Instead of an ongoing war between the sexes, there can be mutually enhancing relationships between men and women.

11
APPRECIATING SENSUALITY

How pleasurable is a hug? A kiss? A caress? If you are like most men, you rate these activities fairly low on the scale of things that are essential to your happiness.

You didn't always feel that way. In fact, when you were a baby your attitudes were quite different. Your need for affection was as vital for you as the food you ate or the air you breathed. And if you had suddenly been deprived of physical tenderness, the effect would have been almost as devastating as the absence of food or oxygen. It is a scientific fact that babies do not develop normally and sometimes become ill if they are not regularly given physical warmth and affection. To an infant, the physical expression of love is essential nourishment. A major cause of the "failure to thrive" phenomenon in young children is the lack of touching and affection.

It isn't difficult to put oneself in the place of an infant and to imagine why this need should exist. To a baby, physical affection, besides being a source of pleasure, means that it is being protected, cared for. To a certain extent, we outgrow this need and develop the capacity to be reassured through means other than physical ones. To an older child, a smile or a kind word may have the same effect as a physical display of affection. And yet we never entirely lose our need for physical warmth and tenderness, nor should we. Whether we are eight or eighty, it is nice to be touched.

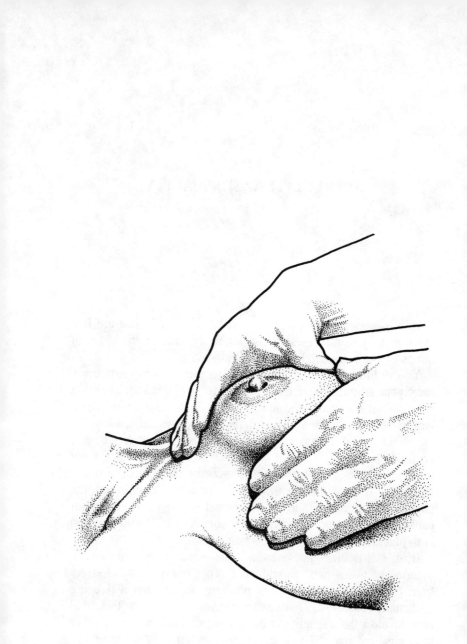

Erotic touching and massaging can be considered non-goal-oriented pleasure and a source of rewarding physical contact.

TOUCH DEPRIVATION IN MALES

Unfortunately, as men grow older, we seem to touch and be touched less and less. Studies have shown that from a very early age, boys are treated with far less physical affection than girls. Such sexual differentiation is part of society's campaign to make us strong, tough, self-reliant, even stoic, to prepare us for the rigors of adult male competition. Frankly, there is little or no evidence to support this type of male training program. The side effects of this deprivation have a negative effect on adult male sexuality.

There is a strong tendency for males to regard nearly all sexual situations as basically competitive and goal-oriented. In his relations with women, the man is encouraged to seek the goal of intercourse. The man who "scores" with a woman is regarded with admiration by his male friends, and the one who scores with many women is accorded special respect and envy. In the sexual interaction itself, the goal is orgasm; this brief, intense sensation is considered by most males to be the only really worthwhile part of sex. The average man achieves orgasm rather quickly—usually within two to five minutes after intromission. Even when he learns to prolong the experience, he does so for the benefit of his female partner, whose responses are usually not as quick as his own. As for the physical expressions of affection that precede intercourse, the very name that has been given to them—foreplay—conveys the idea that they are something of lesser importance, mere preliminaries leading up to the "real thing."

This tendency to sell short all experiences other than orgasm is related to our early training, to the fact that males are encouraged to do without physical expressions of affection. This early learning has convinced us to dismiss kisses, hugs, and spontaneous caresses as having little value if they are not followed by intercourse and orgasm. We tend to forget that such experiences can be highly pleasurable in themselves. The fact that women place a higher value on nongoal-oriented pleasuring reflects in part the greater freedom they are permitted in the physical expression of affection as children and adults. This disparity between the values that men and women place on physical affection and sensuality is frequently a source of contention and misunderstanding between couples.

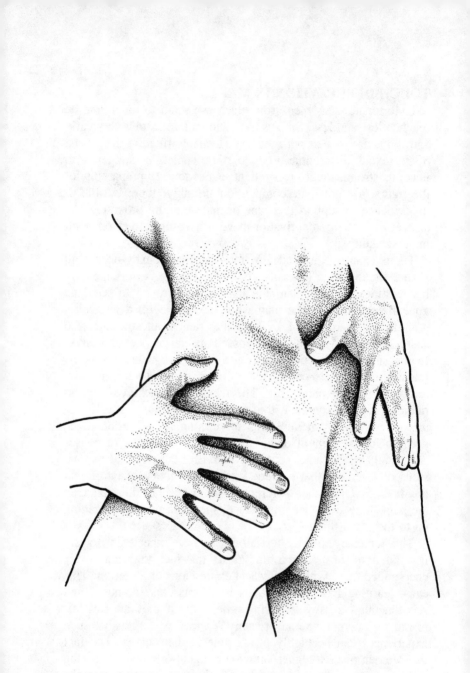

Caressing and firm grasping can convey the familiar sense of security and comfort we enjoyed as children.

MALE-FEMALE TOUCHING

It is common for women to express dissatisfaction with the amount of intimate contact and physical affection they receive from their partners—both inside and outside the bedroom. Men are often confused by this criticism because it is difficult for them to think of affection and/or sensuality as being particularly enjoyable or worthwhile. They tend to regard the expression of physical love as a specialized activity that is circumscribed spatially by the four walls of the bedroom and temporally by the time between lights-out and sleep. The touching that occurs is goal-oriented (intercourse and orgasm).

The truth is, we have imposed on ourselves a state of sensual impoverishment. By opening ourselves to the possibilities of nongoal-oriented pleasure, we can regain the rich and rewarding world of spontaneous physical affection. Affectionate touching can convey not only the sense of protection, security, and comfort that we enjoyed as children but also adult emotions such as respect, gratitude, and sexual attraction. As well as providing a heightened sense of physical pleasure, the development of sensual awareness can have a positive effect on a couple's emotional and sexual relationship. It is a skill well worth learning.

Many men would define sexual pleasure as the enjoyable sensations experienced through the genitals during intercourse. This definition is an extremely narrow one since it eliminates all the nongenital pleasures that we experience during sex. For example, what about the pleasure of seeing our partner's body, either nude or in various stages of undress? What of the pleasure of whispered words of love, or the excitement of hearing our partner's moans and breathing? What of the smell of our partner's body mingling with our own? What of the sense of movement as we engage in coital thrusting? What of the tastes experienced during oral-genital sex? What of the myriad number of ways in which one human being can pleasurably stroke and caress another?

Nor is sensual pleasure by any means limited to the bedroom. For example, there is the exquisite thrill of touching knees under a table. There is the erotic reaction we have to sniffing a particular perfume in the street or in an elevator. And there are the peculiar pelvic sensations we may experience in response to a certain word or phrase spoken in a certain tone of voice. If we are honest with ourselves, it becomes obvious that we can be sensual and sexual people twenty-four hours a day, that pleasure may occur anytime, anywhere, and that we can be receptive to it through all our five senses. Thus, we see the folly of trying to limit sex to a strictly delineated time and place (the bedroom at night) and to a specific range of physical sensations (the penis, intercourse, and the three to ten seconds of orgasm). What makes a sensation sexual is the interpretation we place on it and the feelings that result. It is the mind that is the ultimate sex organ, determining what will turn us on and what will turn us off.

PLEASURING AND INTERCOURSE

Unfortunately, this mind of ours too often acts as a censor, closing down pleasurable circuits, forbidding nongoal-oriented feelings. Touching, caressing, and kissing are most exciting at the beginning of a relationship because the couple has shared relatively few of these experiences, and hopes for more intensity. Each person is learning how the other expresses his or her affection, and each anticipates further sensual exploration.

Discovering new things about one's partner can be a stimulating and exciting experience. For couples who have not yet had intercourse, the fantasies about it are often rich and varied. But as a couple becomes increasingly involved sexually, and begins to have intercourse regularly, simple gestures of affection often lose their significance. Intercourse, enjoyed on a regular basis, tends to become the primary or sole means of displaying physical affection. Kissing and caressing, once so exciting and important, now become mere "foreplay," a brief, hurried prelude to coitus. What began as nondemanding, pleasure-oriented touching gives way to goal-oriented arousal for intercourse.

While there is no disputing the fact that intercourse is the ultimate in sexual expression, there is something very wrong with the idea that other sensual and affectionate behavior is worth engaging in only when it is followed by intercourse. In fact, if intercourse is to continue to be exciting and satisfying, there must be experimentation, spontaneity, and variety. Trying new intercourse positions, of which there are dozens, is one way of introducing novelty into the sexual relationship. But there are countless ways of expressing affection through behavior that does not necessarily lead to intercourse. If we want to introduce new energy and enjoyment into our sex lives, what better way than to concentrate on reopening our closed circuits, expanding our consciousness to include modes of sensuality that we have allowed to fall into disuse, and thus opening up a whole new world of sexual experiences? Sometimes this can lead to intercourse and orgasm, and at other times it can be a way of communicating pleasure, playfulness, or sensuality for itself.

One of the main reasons we lose our capacity to experience pleasure freely and spontaneously is that we have allowed ourselves to become too damned grown-up. As children, we responded intensely to the world because each experience was new and we allowed ourselves to be curious and involved ourselves completely in the experience. But as we matured, we became absorbed by our responsibilities. We assumed that our knowledge of the world was complete and that we knew all there was to know, especially sexually. If we could recapture that openness of mind and senses, we would find that the world is still full of novel and surprising experiences. The number of ways of experiencing physical affection is almost limitless, and, of course, part of the fun is discovering new activities that are pleasurable and exciting. Here are some guidelines other men and couples have utilized to apply new elements of affection and sensuality to their relationships.

Sensuality Guidelines

Learn to concentrate on and to increase your awareness of ordinary acts of physical touching such as hand contact. Pick up your partner's hand and spend some moments examining it as though you are seeing it for the first time. Tenderly explore each aspect, allowing yourself to focus on tiny details—the nails, the cuticles, the knuckles, the loose folds of skin between the fingers, the veins on the back of the hand. Turn her hand over and trace the lines of the palm with your fingertip. Be aware of the delicate tactile messages that you are sending to your partner through this contact.

Set aside some time for sensual exploration, or you might be more comfortable doing this spontaneously. If the latter, your partner may be initially surprised by your attentions, particularly if you are not in the habit of acting this way. But provided that you are genuinely tender and affectionate, it is likely she will be pleased and responsive. In fact, the pleasant surprise caused by a spontaneous act of affection often enhances its impact and may serve to trigger the release of sexual feelings, the intensity of which can be quite startling.

The eyes can be organs of sensual communication. In everyday life, we observe strict rules about the amount and type of eye contact permissible with other individuals. Allowing ourselves to gaze long and deeply into another person's eyes can be an experience of special intimacy. Prolonged eye contact may be combined with other forms of affectionate expression such as touching, caressing, and hand-holding. This can serve to create a moment filled with poignant and romantic sensuality.

A back rub or a massage is another way of expressing affection as well as a pleasant, relaxing experience for your partner. It is an excellent method of projecting a sense of caring and of promoting relaxed, comfortable feelings. Massage can be even more enjoyable if both of you are nude. In fact, this is an especially comfortable way to experience nudity in a nonintercourse situation. The point of a physical massage is to relax the muscles of the body through kneading, pressing, and stretching motions. If you like, you can learn the fine points of massage—the special movements designed to relax specific parts of the musculature. Consult the various books available, or you could even take a course in the subject—preferably you and your partner together.

Sensual massage focuses on nondemand, comfortable, pleasure-oriented feelings between you and your partner. Try to make your touching slow, rhythmic, and tender, with no demand for response other than the experience of pleasure. One way of making sensual massage even more enjoyable is to use a scented oil (or baby oil, body lotion, or powder) as a lubricant. It is most satisfying if both partners learn to do massage. You can integrate massage into your life so that either of you can ask for a sensual body massage without feeling self-conscious. Besides being relaxing, enjoyable, and invigorating, massage is an excellent way of becoming at ease and familiar with your partner's body and of learning about sensual communication in ways that can be beneficial to sexual functioning. You can't go wrong if you use your hands sensitively and gently and if you're open to responses about what feels good.

Another highly pleasurable experience is to bathe or shower with your partner. If you are not in the habit of doing this, there may be some embarrassment and discomfort the first time you try it. Most of us think of bathing as a solitary activity, and while the idea of doing it with a partner may be appealing, there is an initial awkwardness. Try suggesting it to your partner casually. For example, the next time she takes a bath, you might say, "Do you mind if I join you?" If your partner has a splitting headache and wants to spend a quiet hour in a warm tub, your best bet would be to accept a no and see if she'd be open to this at another time. If the initial negative response seems to be based more on self-consciousness, you might try countering by saying, "Come on, it'll be fun," or "We don't have to do anything except enjoy a bath together." Showering or bathing is a sensual, relaxing experience and a nice way of exploring new possibilities of touching. You can take turns slowly soaping each other. The addition of warm water and rich, soapy lather enhances the feeling of caressing your partner's body. You can extend the pleasure of this experience by slowly and caringly drying each other. Brushing your partner's hair is another way of turning a commonplace, personal act into a shared sensual experience. Showering or bathing together can be an excellent preparation for mutual pleasuring and intercourse because it is a wonderful way of becoming relaxed and open to physical sensations. And it has the advantage of making the body clean and sweet-smelling so that it is a particular pleasure both to touch and be touched.

Steve

Steve thought of himself as a "new man," liberated from the restraints of the traditional male role. He'd been married five years to Susan, and they had a two-year-old daughter. Steve was a very involved parent. However, because there were many practical time demands, sex became the thing they did late at night after their child was asleep. Although both Steve and Susan were playful and affectionate with their daughter, they had fallen into a pattern where they were not very affectionate with each other. One night they had a fire in the fireplace, and their child curled up and fell asleep. As Steve and Susan were basking in the glow of the fire, Steve became aware of how much he missed these kinds of experiences. As a premarital couple, and early in their marriage, they had been a very affectionate and playful couple. Both looked back fondly on their courtship, when they would cuddle on the couch for an hour; shower together and even be sexual in the shower; engage in long, sensual touching sessions that usually culminated in intercourse; and go out of their way to exchange hugs. Steve reflected on and shared with Susan how disappointed he was that they had allowed this aspect of their lives to wither.

Steve was surprised when she challenged his assumption that it had to be that way. They put their daughter to bed and returned to the fire. Steve found the next hour and a half the most enjoyable of the past year. They talked, hugged, caressed, recalled memories, and thoroughly enjoyed a very sensuous time. It eventually culminated in intercourse since both were very sexually aroused. However, even if they had stayed with sensual play, it would have been a very worthwhile experience.

The next day Steve and Susan went for a walk and vowed that they would rebuild sensuality in their marriage. They realized the prior night had been a special experience that would not be easily duplicated, but they could engage in touching both inside and outside the bedroom as a way of reaffirming their caring and love for each other. Being affectionate with each other was a vital part of their life that had slipped away and seemed even more important now as they strove to recapture it. In addition, they began doing whole-family hugs. Steve realized that sexuality was more than late-night intercourse. He valued their affectionate and sensual time as a way of keeping contact and building sexual anticipation.

OTHER FUNCTIONS OF TOUCH

Although most instances of sensual and sexual expression are to convey a message of caring, affection, and tenderness, this need not always be the case. Many healthy relationships have a degree of frustration or tension built into them, and it is better to express such feelings in a playful, physical way rather than to let them fester inside us. There are many ways we can do this, such as having a pillow fight or a wrestling or tickling match. Sometimes, when giving your partner a massage, you may want to bear down hard or rub rapidly. Expressing tensions and frustrations in these ways can be stimulating sexually as well as provide an emotional release.

Couples can feel free to express themselves in ways that might seem childish or foolish. You might try playing artificial roles, indulging in fantasy and pantomime. Some of the more common roles include the princess and the slave, the sultan and the harem girl, and the adventurer and the shy, naive person. These are just a few of the possibilities. The fact that both you and your partner recognize that these are fantasies and not reality can allow you to express yourself freely and to give vent to feelings and attitudes that you ordinarily avoid and may even disapprove of in real life. Touch can serve a number of emotional functions in a relationship.

ADDING AFFECTION AND SENSUALITY TO YOUR LIFE

These are just a few of the many ways available for developing your sensual awareness and adding new excitement and meaning to your relationship. The situations in which we are apt to experience sensual or sexual feelings are potentially unlimited. Imagination, sensitivity, and a willingness to try new activities are the qualities we can strive for to expand our pleasure quotient. There is little doubt that bringing greater sensuality to your relationship will have a positive effect on the quality of your sex life. But the pleasure to be derived from introducing spontaneous, novel, affectionate, and sensual experiences into a relationship is a substantial reward in its own right.

12

PLEASURING, INTERCOURSE, AFTERGLOW

I've always thought it odd that people should consider it a compliment to a man's sexual prowess to compare him with certain male animals—a bull, a stallion, a billy goat, or a rooster—or to describe him as a "stud." The truth is that most animals are not very good lovers.

Anyone who has spent time on a farm is probably well acquainted with the mating habits of roosters. The male bird spends his time strutting about, surrounded by his flock of hens, pecking at the ground and every so often giving out with a strident call of pure, mindless self-affirmation. When the urge strikes him, he will pursue one of the hens and mount her. After a few seconds of rapid thrusting, he ejaculates, and it is all over. The hen moves off to continue her search for bugs while the rooster ruffles his feathers and chortles with satisfaction. True, he repeats this performance several dozen times a day, a feat that no human male could duplicate. But what is the good of such sexual capacity if it means settling for a total lack of variety and intimacy in sex?

The mating behavior of the rooster is completely instinctive. Its purpose is simply to produce more fowl, and it serves this purpose quite well. It never occurs to either the hen or the rooster that there should be anything more to sex; they haven't got the brains to realize they are missing anything. And so they keep on having intercourse in the same old way, giving birth to more hens and roosters.

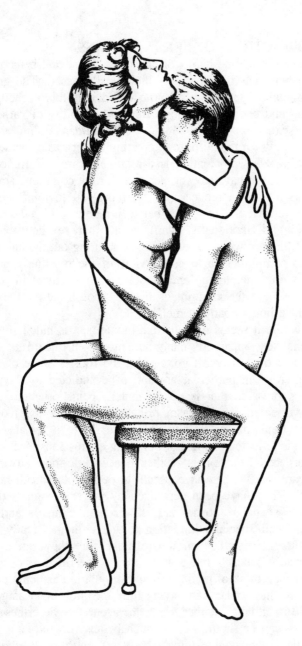

One of many creative positions for intercourse. Such creativity leads to savoring and prolonging the experience rather than rushing frenziedly to orgasm.

THE FUNCTIONS OF SEX IN HUMANS

Unlike the mating habits of chickens, the sexual behavior of human beings is only partially biologically based. The greater part of human sexuality is learned, and it is this capacity for learning and choice that allows for the possibility of variety in human sexual expression. Moreover, we humans do not engage in sex purely for the purpose of creating duplicates of ourselves. In fact, sex for procreation is a relatively rare occurrence for most of us. We have sex for pleasure, for the communication of love, as a tension reducer, for warmth, and to reinforce and deepen intimacy. Thus, sex between humans is a far more complex and emotionally significant act than sex between animals. Although we use the phrase ''You bring out the animal in me'' to compliment a lover, in view of the peculiarly human capacity for imagination and emotional involvement in sex, it would be a greater compliment to say, ''You bring out the most passionate human parts of me.''

But while it seems obvious that human sex is much superior to animal sex, apparently many humans haven't heard the news yet. Some of us haven't gotten past the rooster stage of love-making. Men in particular are apt to be addicted to a type of sexual expression that is goal oriented, penis oriented, intercourse oriented, and orgasm oriented. Many of us, like the rooster, think of sex as something we do to a female. This attitude is reflected in some of our slang expressions, such as ''I laid her'' or ''I made her.'' Other men, a little more advanced, are aware that women have a right to derive pleasure from sex as well. They have been persuaded by the sex manuals that a woman's sexual responses are slower than a man's and that women need special stimulation to make them ''ready'' for intercourse. So, it is their job to make sure they ''give their partner an orgasm''—like a work order to be filled.

Most men think of nonintercourse stimulation as being exclusively for the woman and having little meaning or pleasure for them. But actually, neither *to* nor *for* accurately describes what sexuality can or should be. A much better word is *with*. Both the male body and the female body are enormously complex structures, gloriously endowed with the capacity to experience pleasure. The most satisfying sexual expression is a cooperative enterprise in which two people not only give each other pleasure but guide the partner to share what is most pleasureable and arousing. This sharing, this sensual and sexual give-and-take, is the essence of human sexuality. It is the quality that distinguishes our sexual behavior from the blind, instinctive demands of the animal kingdom.

MALE AND FEMALE SIMILARITIES AND DIFFERENCES

Male and female sexual responses have many more similarities than differences. Men and women need to think of each other as sexual persons equally able to experience desire, arousal, orgasm, and emotional satisfaction from sexuality. But there is a major difference that must be understood: female sexual response is more variable and complex—not necessarily better or worse—than that of the male. The woman may be nonorgasmic, singly orgasmic, or multiorgasmic, and this can occur during any phase of the sexual experience. The male typically has a single orgasm, which ocurs during intercourse.

The title of this chapter—"Pleasuring, Intercourse, Afterglow"—is meant to emphasize the fact that there is more to sex than just "getting it in and getting it off." Intercourse—that part of sex between intromission and ejaculation—may be the high point, but it is not the be-all and end-all of sexuality. It is, rather, one of the many activities in which partners give each other pleasure. Intercourse can be even more rewarding if we allow ourselves to freely explore and enjoy the range of sensual and sexual expression surrounding it. In fact, intercourse might best be conceptualized as simply another pleasuring technique, a special and integral one but not separate from the pleasuring experience.

In this chapter, we will consider pleasuring, intercourse, and afterglow as three separate aspects of sex. Each phase is characterized by its own distinct feelings as well as by some that are common to all three. Each can be enjoyable in its own right, for its own sake, as well as be part of the complete sexual experience. The three phases may be enjoyed in different combinations, depending on the feelings of the couple and on the limitations imposed by the external situation. For example, pleasuring may lead into intercourse, or it may be engaged in

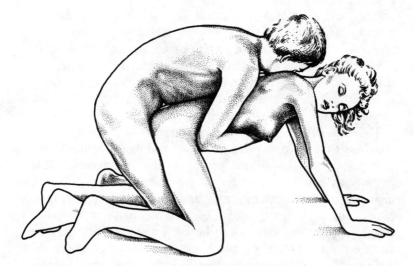

One of many positions for sexual intercourse. All too often
only one position is employed during a session of lovemaking.

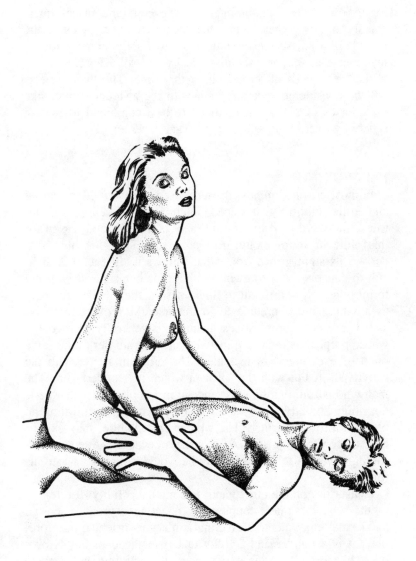

The woman astride the man while both continue caressing each other. This can be considered "pleasuring" as much as intercourse.

for its own sake without intercourse ever taking place. Intercourse, on the other hand, may begin at once, without the prelude of a pleasuring session. Afterglow activities may follow intercourse or they may be dispensed with—all according to the wishes and needs of the couple at that time. The three aspects will be considered separately but with the awareness that, like the courses of a fine meal, they are best combined to form a satisfying overall emotional and sexual experience.

PLEASURING

In most peoples' minds, the term used to describe the sensual and erotic activities that precede intercourse is *foreplay*. I prefer to use the word *pleasuring*, and there is a very good reason for this shift in terminology. *Foreplay* suggests something that derives its significance from what follows it. Just as it is difficult to conceive of a foreword without the book that it is meant to introduce, it is difficult to think of something called foreplay as anything but a prelude to intercourse. Moreover, foreplay, as it is presented in most sex manuals, is generally a procedure whose purpose is to arouse the woman, to bring her to the same pitch of excitement as the man. The problem is not with the activity itself but with the spirit in which it is undertaken. The man who is told that he must engage in foreplay feels that he is not doing something for his own enjoyment but is fulfilling an obligation to his partner. The woman, meanwhile, may experience discomfort and self-consciousness because she feels she is forcing the man to do something he would rather not waste his time on.

Pleasuring, on the other hand, is a mutual activity. It refers to all the behaviors that a couple may engage in to produce sensual and sexual enjoyment. Pleasuring is not goal-oriented like foreplay; it is a nondemand activity that is engaged in for its own sake. In most pleasuring experiences, the activities will lead to more and more arousal and will eventually culminate in intercourse. But this need not be so. Pleasuring experiences that are not followed by intercourse can be particularly erotic and tantalizing. Emily and I have found that an occasional session of pleasuring—say, every month or two—in which we agree beforehand not to proceed to intercourse, no matter how turned on we become, provides an excellent way of reexploring our erotic responses and of retaining variety and novelty in our sexual relationship.

Pleasuring can be particularly important for men since most of us pay little attention to the nuances of our feelings. We are well acquainted with the pleasure of orgasm, but we are often unaware of what else can make us feel good. We have a tendency to rate the value of our sexual responses in terms of intensity, and since orgasm is the most intense physical sensation we have experienced, we are orgasm-oriented. But the intensity of a sensation depends to a great extent on how well attuned to it we are. When we learn to increase our sensitivity to the range of sensual and sexual feelings other than orgasm, the intensity of these sensations will increase in our perception. In order to develop this sensitivity, we need to change our approach to sex. We need to accept that there is more to a man's body than just a penis, that there is more to sex than intercourse, and that there is more to sexuality than the three to ten seconds of orgasm. Once you make this change, you will find that developing awareness of a broader range of sensual stimuli is one of the best favors you can do for yourself. And, of course, the effect of this heightened sensitivity on your relationship will be extremely beneficial.

Nongoal Orientation

Probably the most difficult concept for most men to comprehend in relation to pleasuring is the nongoal orientation. Pleasuring need not lead to intercourse and orgasm. It is common for men (and women) to place an implicit demand on themselves and their sex partners that every affectionate or erotic encounter must culminate in intercourse. For many men, the fulfillment of this requirement becomes a matter of pride, a test of their masculinity. Thus, when a particular sexual encounter does not end in intercourse, they may feel that there is something wrong with them. Or they may consider nondemand, nongoal-oriented sex play as somehow immature, reminiscent of the sessions of necking and petting they experienced as adolescents. But if you are honest with yourself, you will remember that you enjoyed those sessions very much. There is no reason why you shouldn't enjoy them again, perhaps even more so, since your greater maturity as well as the comfort of a stable relationship allow you to introduce much greater intimacy and experimentation into nongoal-oriented pleasuring. We feel that the consummation of each sexual encounter with intercourse and orgasm is a special privilege we have earned by becoming adults. What we forget is that true maturity means freedom, the right to choose, the ability to be self-directing. The mature person can choose not to press for intercourse in a particular sexual experience, or he or she can choose to experience orgasm through manual or oral-genital stimulation.

Pleasuring Experiences

The varieties of pleasuring techniques are endless, but here are some suggestions drawn from my own experience and the experience of helping couples in sex therapy. If you and your partner decide to devote time specifically to learning techniques of pleasuring, be sure to give yourselves at least half an hour free of interruptions. Take the phone off the hook. Make whatever preparations you like to set the mood. Turn the lights in your bedroom down if you wish (but not off—you'll want to see what you're doing), or light a candle. You might want to put a favorite record on the stereo or burn some incense. Emily and I have a scented candle in our bedroom that seems to create just the right sensual atmosphere for us, but the choice of such paraphernalia depends entirely on individual tastes.

An excellent way to structure your pleasuring is to designate one partner as the giver and the other as the recipient. These roles are arbitrary and might be determined by flipping a coin. The role of the recipient is to accept pleasure passively. You will probably find this a great deal harder than it sounds. When you are the recipient, try closing your eyes during the experience. This will make it easier for you to concentrate on your own sensations and will cut down on whatever self-consciousness you or your partner may feel. The giver's role is to actively give pleasure and to explore and learn about the partner's body. The first time you might want to focus on only nongenital touching, the idea being to explore sensual as opposed to sexual stimulation. The giver can be aware of his or her own sensations and responses as he or she gives stimulation. The recipient needs to be receptive to a wide variety of sensual experiences to discover what is most comfortable and pleasuring. The giver can feel free to use both hard and light massage, just barely touching with the fingertips, kissing, licking, biting, or any other technique the giver might find enjoyable.

Switch at some point during the session so that each partner gets a chance to experience both roles. Many couples find that their learning is facilitated when they begin with a clear structure. As they become more comfortable with the pleasuring concepts and techniques, the process becomes more mutual and interactive, and less structured.

You might begin with the recipient lying facedown. The giver can then stroke and caress the partner from head to toe, experimenting with different kinds of touching, kissing, massaging, all the while being aware of the look and feel of the various parts of the body. Later, the recipient can turn over and the giver can continue touching and exploring the front of the body. Remember to begin your pleasuring sessions with nongenital touching and to proceed in later sessions to stimulating the genitals and breasts. Many men are highly sensitive in the breast and nipple area; you may not have been aware of this because you have been misinformed that only the woman's breast is an "erogenous zone." Although looking at your partner's body is an important part of pleasuring, an interesting variation of the pleasuring method is for both partners to keep their eyes shut. This has the effect of heightening your other senses and of making you aware of feelings you might miss otherwise.

Those couples who have not engaged extensively in pleasuring activities may be somewhat ignorant of one another's sexual anatomy. For example, many men who are aware that the clitoris is a particularly sensitive area may not realize that direct clitoral stimulation can be unpleasant and even painful. It is generally more effective to apply stimulation around the clitoral shaft and inner lips (labia minora). Let your partner guide you, as she is the expert on her own sexual responses.

In subsequent pleasuring sessions, the recipient can participate more actively by putting his or her hands over those of the partner and guiding to areas that are particularly sensitive. Show the partner the particular kind of touch that is most arousing by using your hand over hers to guide her. This type of nonverbal guidance is particularly important and effective. Sometimes the difference between a pleasant and an unpleasant sensation may be a fraction of an inch to the right or left or a bit more or less pressure. A very effective way to give such guidance is through touch. During later sessions, both partners can keep their eyes open and use visual contact to communicate affection and responsiveness. If something the partner does produces discomfort, the recipient should not call a halt, but rather suggest some alternative activity. By the same token, if the giver notices stress or uneasiness in the partner, he or she shouldn't stop, but should rather go back to a previous activity that was more comfortable. In this way, negative response can be incorporated into the couple's interaction without interrupting the atmosphere of receptivity and responsiveness that has been created between them.

There are many positions that are effective for pleasuring—in fact, quite a few more than there are for intercourse. In a particularly satisfying one, the giver sits upright with back against the wall or headboard and legs spread apart, and the recipient sits with back leaning against the giver's chest. This position not only allows the giver full access to the partner's body, but it also makes it easy for the recipient to guide the giver's hands to those parts of the body that are particularly sensitive and to demonstrate the kind of touch that is most effective.

Pleasuring activities can be enhanced through the use of emollients such as baby oil, hand lotion, or powder. You could go to a speciality shop and choose a lotion that is nonallergenic and has a smell and texture you like. In fact, you can use anything that your imagination suggests so long as it is stimulating and fun for both of you and not physically harmful. External devices—anything from a vibrator to a feather—are interesting to experiment with.

One thing to remember about pleasuring is that getting an erection need not be interpreted as a sign that pleasuring should be ended and intercourse begun. When an erection occurs during pleasuring, be aware of it, enjoy it, but do not feel that you are obligated to do anything about it. Nor, on the other hand, should you feel alarmed if you do not get an erection. I think of pleasuring as an exercise in whole-body stimulation and response. In these terms, the penis is just a part of the big sex organ known as the human body.

INTERCOURSE

There is no sharp dividing line between pleasuring and intercourse. Pleasuring does not stop when intercourse starts. Many kinds of pleasuring, such as kissing, caressing, breast stimulation, clitoral stimulation, and testicle stimulation, can continue during intercourse. In fact, intercourse itself is really the ultimate form of pleasuring. It is an activity in which a couple gives each other pleasure through the intromission and movement of the penis in the vagina while continuing other stimulation (i.e., multiple stimulation) during intercourse.

Thinking about intercourse in this way can be an eye-opening experience. Studies have shown that the average intercourse experience lasts for between two to five minutes, and orgasm takes up only three to ten seconds of that time. For many males, intercourse has become a mad rush to reach the peak, orgasm. Not that such an intercourse style is necessarily bad. An occasional frenzied "quickie" can be highly exciting and satisfying. However, when "quickies" constitute the entirety of a couple's sexual repertoire, the result is usually monotony, frustration, and eventually resentment on the woman's part. If, on the other hand, a man learns to take his time, to savor the intercourse experience in a leisurely manner, he will find, first, that there are a thousand nuances of pleasure to be enjoyed along the way and, second, that his orgasm is still waiting faithfully for him at the end of the line—and usually better than ever after the slow, tantalizing buildup.

The average man thinks of his pattern of sexual arousal as a steady increase to orgasm, and that is the way it has traditionally been experienced. Actually, though, there are four phases in the sexual arousal cycle: excitement, plateau, orgasm, and resolution. In the first, or excitement, phase, the penis becomes erect and the testes are elevated. If stimulation continues, the male enters the second, or plateau, phase, where his excitement increases, his erection becomes firmer, his breathing becomes heavier, his skin may break out in a "sex flush," and he may begin sweating. Usually intercourse itself begins either at the end of the excitement phase or sometime during the plateau phase. Most males are used to going to intercourse on their first erection, although that is not necessarily the best pattern. The intensity of stimulation (both physical and psychological) is what determines the man's experience of arousal. If he is consistently stimulated, without pause, he might well progress through the excitement and plateau phases and reach the point of ejaculation in a short time, perhaps in a minute or two. If, however, variations in the amount and intensity of stimulation are introduced, then corresponding variations in the pattern of arousal are possible.

Prolonging Intercourse

How can you introduce these variations? What can you do to prolong the experience of intercourse? There are some common folk remedies for rapid ejaculation, such as biting down hard on the corner of the pillow or fixing your mind on something unpleasant and nonsexual such as your income tax payment. These methods might actually be effective in temporarily reducing the intensity of stimulation, but at what cost? Certainly the feeling of a pillow between your teeth or the thought of your tax debts adds nothing positive to the intercourse experience. And using these methods might cause you to build up a sense of resentment against your partner, feeling you are depriving yourself of pleasure for her sake. It also could cause your arousal to decrease and the beginning of erection problems.

Luckily, however, there is a much better way of achieving ejaculatory control. The first step in prolonging intercourse is to discard the demand for quick orgasm. This may seem to be more easily said than done, but there is an established psychological principle you can use to achieve this. The human mind can be fully occupied with only one thought or sensation at any one time. If your attention is fixed on something besides the demand for orgasm, then that demand subsides. It makes far more sense to choose a pleasant focus than an unpleasant one, and the most pleasant focus, as well as the most effective one, is the stimulation you are experiencing at that particular moment. The more fully you concentrate on the sensations of intercourse and are comfortable in the nuances of pleasure you are experiencing, the less intense will be your demand for orgasm, the longer the experience will last, and the more pleasurable it will be.

The difference in approach is roughly that between a sprinter straining to reach the finish line and a person strolling at a leisurely pace through a lovely, enthralling countryside and using all his senses to take in as much of the experience as he can. Enjoy the journey as well as the arrival.

The man has to learn to recognize his point of ejaculatory inevitability, the point at which he loses voluntary control and will ejaculate, no matter what. If you can learn to identify this point, then you can reduce the amount of stimulation of the penis before the point is reached and thereby allow the intercourse experience to last so that it is more enjoyable for you and your partner.

Variety in Positions

Variety is important in intercourse. Of the many possible positions for intercourse, most couples use the male-on-top position exclusively or almost exclusively. There is nothing wrong with this position: it is comfortable, intromission is fairly easy, the penis seldom slips out, and, since the partners face one another, it allows them to kiss and caress each other freely. Other positions, however, offer advantages just as great, and there is no reason to consider the male-on-top position more natural or basic than any other.

The point of trying a variety of positions is not to prove yourself a sexual contortionist or to show that you are not afraid of exotic sexual practices. Rather, it is to introduce a sense of novelty and discovery, which is as important in sex as it is in other aspects of life. Discovering and sharing a new restaurant, a new hobby, a new friend, a new book or movie, or a new way of making love are all experiences that enrich and deepen a couple's feelings. Just as rigidity and monotony can have a deadly effect on a couple's enjoyment of other activities, it can also have a dampening influence on their sex life, eventually making it seem like something kept up primarily out of habit or duty.

Since this book is not meant to be a sex manual, I will not attempt to describe the many other possible positions for intercourse, the most common of which are female-on-top, side-by side, and rear entry. The reader can refer to *Sexual Awareness: Sharing Sexual Pleasure*, which I wrote with Emily, for a variety of pleasuring and intercourse positions and techniques. It is important to emphasize that for optimal sexual pleasure a couple ought to feel free to experiment with positions they have not tried before and to choose those they find particularly comfortable and stimulating. You may find that there are two or three positions that become your favorites and that you use time and time again. There may be others that require a particular mood and that you utilize only on occasion. There may be still others you use rarely, when you are feeling especially adventurous. But you will never build up this repertoire unless you make a special effort to experiment and to find out which positions suit you and which do not.

You can also introduce variety in the type of coital thrusting. Many men rely primarily on a rapid in-and-out thrusting movement in which they control the rhythm. You might want to experiment with a more circular or up-and-down movement, or with a slow, tantalizing rhythm or a rhythm that gradually increases in tempo and then holds steady. The woman can set the tempo for the coital thrusting, rather than the male always controlling it. You could also try a minimal, slow movement (the "quiet vagina" exercise) for a period of time to enjoy the feelings of vaginal containment.

Another element where variety is important is that of who makes the first move. In our male-dominant society, it is usually the man who initiates a sexual encounter. But there is no rational reason why this pattern should be accepted as the norm. There are times in the relationship of any couple when a reversal of the traditional roles can be a turn-on for both partners. In fact, the most satisfying relationship is one in which both partners feel free to initiate and both feel free to say no. The key is for the man to develop a relaxed, positive attitude toward accepting pleasure. In this way he can encourage his partner to express herself in initiating sexual contact and intercourse.

Just as there are times when you experience such urgent sexual desire that you feel almost like devouring your partner as

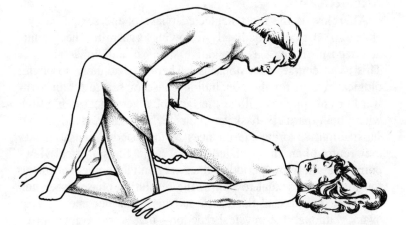

"Pleasuring"—a more felicitous word than foreplay because it better suggests the idea of continuity—does not stop when intercourse begins.

though she were a sumptuous meal, there are doubtless times when she feels the same way about you. You should not be shocked or intimidated by this, but accept and enjoy it. Some men worry about whether they will be able to be turned on and have an erection when their partner initiates. A female initiation is not a demand for immediate erection and intercourse but an invitation for sexual pleasuring that will result in arousal, erection, and intercourse. If the man is not aroused or interested in intercourse at that time, he can say no and suggest another pleasuring activity. Remember, sexuality and intercourse are for pleasure, not performance.

AFTERGLOW

Afterglow is the most neglected phase of the sexual experience. The period immediately following orgasm has been characterized in the past as a negative state, an anticlimactic time. This is, of course, utter nonsense. There is absolutely no physiological reason for the concluding phase of sex to be an awkward or unhappy one. It can, in fact, be a very pleasurable time when both partners bask in their feelings of relaxation and satisfaction, savoring the nuances of their bodily sensations as they return to an unstimulated state. From a physiological viewpoint, the afterglow period is the experiential component of the fourth stage of sexual response, the resolution phase, when the man's sexual arousal decreases and his penis becomes flaccid again. Although the physical reaction—that is, the erect penises becoming flaccid—occurs rather quickly, the entire resolution phase actually takes up a considerable amount of time. In a young man, the vasocongestion of the tissues in the genital area may take three to four hours to disappear completely; in an older man, the period is about a half hour.

Most men assume that intercourse is over with orgasm and that the only possible activities to engage in afterward are to get up and go about their business or to fall asleep. The first pattern may be the result of early experiences with clandestine lovemaking, when it was important to quickly erase all evidence of intercourse for fear of discovery. The second pattern is probably a conditioned response based on the mistaken notion that intercourse is a highly taxing activity and that a man needs to sleep afterward in order to recuperate. Indeed, when intercourse takes place late at night, it may be perfectly acceptable to go to sleep afterward. There is, however, no physiological need to sleep after orgasm, and the man who invariably goes to sleep following intercourse is cheating both himself and his partner of the warm and intimate sharing of sensations and emotions that characterize the afterglow period.

For the woman who is nonorgasmic during intercourse, the afterglow phase provides an opportunity for her partner to manually or orally stimulate her to orgasm. A man must realize that his partner may find it difficult to request additional stimulation and that he should be especially sensitive and responsive to her needs.

One couple I had been treating for sexual dysfunction—a military officer and his wife—provided an excellent example of this problem. The couple had been following a program of pleasuring and had been making rather good progress. The wife had been nonorgasmic during intercourse, however, and her husband had flatly turned down her requests for manual stimulation. We talked about her need during one session, and he agreed, rather reluctantly, that the next time he would try to help bring her to orgasm. But when they next had intercourse, he fell asleep afterward, as usual. Then, remembering his promise, he roused himself and said in a grumpy voice, "Oh, yeah, I almost forgot. Is there anything you want me to do for you now?" The wife became livid. "That's it," she replied. "I'm leaving you!" She did, in fact, leave him, but came back shortly afterward, and the two of them returned to therapy. I concentrated on teaching the husband to be more sensitive to his wife's needs and to view her as an equal sexual person. As his attitude changed, she became more responsive to his touch and eventually became orgasmic both during the pleasuring phase and during afterglow.

Another impediment to a man's enjoyment of the afterglow phase may stem from his feeling that any sort of touching or caressing implies a demand for further sexual activity. There is a physiological phenomenon for males called the "refractory period," when it is physically impossible for a man to respond to sexual stimulation and to get an erection. This period is usually at least fifteen minutes long and can extend to an hour (and longer for an older man). A man may feel that any sort of touching is best avoided during afterglow since it cannot lead to anything. Perhaps he fears that if he fails to respond with an erection, he will be seen as lacking in virility. But if he understands that no further performance is expected of him, he will be able to relax and engage in the nondemand touching, kissing, and holding that makes the afterglow experience such an enjoyable and rewarding one.

Although comfortable tenderness and relaxation are the most common responses during afterglow, other feelings and activities are also possible. As with pleasuring and intercourse, variety, experimentation, and spontaneity in the afterglow period are of prime importance. After orgasm, a couple may find themselves in a playful, happy mood and might express their exuberance by having a glass of wine, taking a shower together, raiding the refrigerator, or taking a walk. As with other phases of sex, optimal satisfaction will result when both partners endeavor to get in touch with their true feelings of the moment and to act on them in a free, spontaneous, and mutually sensitive way.

CLOSING THOUGHTS

If this chapter has had a consistent theme, it is that if a man is open to variation in his sexual experiences, then he will be in a position to discover his sexual likes and dislikes and to choose those activities that are most enjoyable to him. The basic principle of sexual satisfaction is really quite simple. Anything that expands and intensifies a couple's enjoyment of themselves and of each other is good and ought to be encouraged. Anything that limits or nullifies that enjoyment is bad for them (though not necessarily for others) and should be eliminated. The rest is up to you. Sexuality is yours to make of what you will. Why not make the most of it.

13
SEXUAL FANTASIES: YOUR PRIVATE X-RATED CINEMA

The wonderful thing about sexual fantasies is that you can have them any way you like. You and you alone have the last word on casting, plot, direction, editing, camera angles, and special effects. And since you are the only person who ever will or can see your fantasies, you need never be concerned with bad reviews or censorship. As an accompaniment to masturbation, sexual fantasies can be marvelously effective for increasing arousal. A sexual fantasy can provide a pleasant interlude in the middle of a tedious day. During intercourse, fantasy can transform a familiar sex partner into someone exotic, unattainable. In short, every sexual experience that you have ever wanted or wondered about can be yours through the magic of fantasy.

But then why do we suffer so much anxiety, guilt, and confusion because of our sexual fantasies? Why do we worry that our fantasies may be used as evidence to prove us "abnormal" or "perverse"? Why do we fear that our sexual fantasies will someday get out of control, that instead of being mere entertainment, they will begin to exert a sinister influence over our actions in the real world? If there is no such thing as censorship where fantasy is concerned, why do we often feel as though a strike force from the Antismut League were standing outside our head, ready to march in and close us down?

In order to answer these questions, we must explore some of the attitudes our society has held regarding fantasy in general and sexual fantasy in particular.

The major portion of our lives is rational and predictable, proceeding smoothly according to certain agreed-upon rules and conventions. We wake up at the same time each morning, take the same drive or subway ride to work, and interact with our friends and associates using the same conversational formulas. Even when something unexpected happens—a sudden promotion or a traffic accident—there are certain conventional ways of reacting to it (buy a bottle of champagne, get the other fellow's license number and the name of his insurance company). There are individual differences in behavior, and there are moments when we do act spontaneously and unpredictably. But for the most part people spend their day-to-day lives acting according to accepted patterns. Individuals who have no patterns are considered rather odd.

In fantasy, however, all the patterns, all the rules, all the conventions, can be and are overturned. We may fantasize ourselves acting in ways that would be unacceptable or disastrous in daily life. We may insult and humiliate people with whom we are normally restrained and respectful. We may imagine ourselves having sex with people who are unavailable or simply peripheral to our lives: a movie star, a bank teller, our best friend's wife. Moreover, in our fantasies, we frequently perform actions that we would never dream of doing in real life. A mild-mannered person might imagine himself battering an enemy to a pulp; a man might fantasize raping his female boss; a practicing homosexual might imagine himself with a female sex partner. We do not share these fantasies with others, and so, with no basis for comparison, we are apt to think that our own fantasies are far more bizarre than anyone else's. The truth is that the fantasy life of nearly everyone is strange, unpredictable, socially nonacceptable, and chaotic, compared with the ordered, rational events that occur in the everyday world.

The trouble comes when we try to understand our fantasies in the same way we explain our everyday experiences. The attempt fails because fantasies operate outside the system of rational modes of thought. Fantasy experiences have a definite rationale and value in and of themselves.

THE DIFFERENCE BETWEEN
FANTASY AND BEHAVIOR

The way we respond to our fantasies depends largely on cultural and educational backgrounds. In Western cultural tradition, until recently, fantasy has been viewed with considerable apprehension. The Judeo-Christian tradition has always held that a "good" person is good not only in action but also in thought. Thus, "impure" thoughts—especially sexual fantasies— were considered the work of the devil. The New Testament states in no uncertain terms that "whosoever lookest on a woman to lust after her hath committed adultery with her already in his heart." This view got former president Jimmy Carter a lot of bad publicity in his infamous *Playboy* interview. Such an attitude tends to blur the crucially important distinction between thought and action, between fantasy and reality. A far more productive attitude would be one that allowed us to be comfortable with our fantasy life as well as to use it to promote our greater happiness and pleasure.

While few of us still believe that every time we have a sexual fantasy we are under the influence of Satan, there does remain a good deal of confusion about the relationship of fantasy to everyday life. We are unsure whether, or to what extent, our fantasies represent what we actually want to do or are capable of doing. Do a married man's fantasies of having sex with other women mean that he really does not love his wife? Do a man's fantasies of rape mean that he is in danger of committing sexual assault? Do a heterosexual's fantasies of sex with other men mean that he is really a latent homosexual? These are the sort of questions that cause the greatest anxiety for us where fantasy is concerned. We are aware that there is some sort of relationship between fantasy and behavior, but we are unaware of just what that relationship is. How closely does fantasy approach day-to-day existence? To what extent are we responsible for our fantasies?

In dealing with these questions, the primary concept to keep in mind is that there is a profound difference between thinking about doing something and actually doing it. Almost everyone has aggressive, antisocial, and bizarre sexual fantasies at some time or another, but few people ever act out any of these fantasies. The fact is that the worst danger of antisocial fantasies is not that they will be acted out, but rather the guilt feelings they engender. Guilt is a powerful and self-defeating emotion. While sexual fantasies themselves need not have any appreciable effect on a person's behavior, guilt experienced as a result of these fantasies frequently has a strong effect. It can serve as a negative motivating force that keeps a person obsessively focusing on a particular fantasy. It may become strong enough to influence our actual sexual behavior, making us uncomfortable with our sexual feelings or leading us to avoid situations in which the fantasies are suggested. Such feelings of discomfort may distort a person's sexual self-esteem and discourage communication between partners.

In trying to come to terms with our sexual fantasies, we should be concerned not with finding a way to "purify" our thoughts, or to impose some sort of rigid control or limitation on our fantasies, but rather with effectively desensitizing ourselves to the guilt we feel about having fantasies. As we shall see, we can learn to put our fantasies to good use. As for guilt, it has no positive use whatsoever.

MISUSE OF FANTASIES

When a particular thought or idea is associated in our minds with guilt, fear, or anxiety, the thought takes on a power and importance it ordinarily would not have, and we thus have less control over it. In some cases, a single fantasy may assume the central focus in a person's life, displacing other forms of sexual enjoyment. In such cases, the fantasy may produce intense arousal, but also intense guilt—a very unhealthy combination of emotions. For example, a man who has intense and guilt-laden sexual fantasies about little girls, and who becomes obsessed with that one fantasy, is in big trouble. The combination of guilt and compulsion can result in the man's becoming a pedophile (a sexual abuser of children). The fantasy and behavior combine to have a compulsive, addictive quality. Carried to this extreme, obsessive fantasies lead to fetishism, the centering of sexual feelings on some inanimate object, which then becomes the sole stimulus capable of triggering a sexual response. Fetishists are sometimes portrayed humorously as roguish old gentlemen gloating lasciviously over their collections of women's shoes or lace panties. But fetishism is a sad affair in real life, for it represents a severe limitation on the person's emotional and sexual life. A man's obsession with women's underwear is not bad because it is morally wrong; it is bad because it is the only thing he has, because it controls his sexual expression. While fetishism is an extreme form, guilt-laden, obsessive sexual fantasies need to be avoided, not on moral grounds but because they drastically reduce the pleasure we derive from our sexuality and instead cause emotional and sexual problems.

I believe that the best general course to follow, then, with regard to sexual fantasy is not to suppress your erotic imaginings or to reject socially unacceptable fantasies but to deliberately cultivate as widely varied a repertoire as you find enjoyable. To return for a moment to my cinematic metaphor, it makes little sense to watch the same film over and over again when you have at your disposal the enormous resources of a private Hollywood inside your head. The important thing to keep in mind is that whatever erotic entertainments we invent, the vast majority of us are in no danger whatever of behaviorally wandering outside the bounds of normalcy. There is no such thing as an unhealthy sexual fantasy, as long as it remains a fantasy and doesn't become obsessive and acted out in a compulsive, self-defeating manner.

POSITIVE FUNCTIONS OF FANTASY

Not only are sexual fantasies normal and healthy, but they also serve useful purposes. We all need an occasional vacation from the rationality of everyday life, and fantasy provides just that. Dreams—perhaps the most common mode of our fantasy lives—are a case in point. Just about everyone dreams, although many people may not recall having dreamed. In the course of an average night's sleep, two to three hours are spent dreaming. Studies have shown that people deprived of their dreams become irritable and depressed. If the deprivation continues over a period of time, a severe state of psychological disorientation can develop. Dreams provide a nonrational "pressure valve," without which our rational, controlled, waking lives would be stressed.

Perhaps because they intuitively recognize the great importance of dreaming to mental health and psychological well-being, other cultures emphasize the positive elements of dreaming. There is a Malaysian culture that teaches its children how to dream "correctly"; the family members share their dreams each morning, and the parents instruct their children in how they might improve them. But we tend to write off dreams as unimportant unless we are undergoing psychoanalysis, in which case we report them to our analyst. In any event, we do not consider our dreams to be an integral part of our lives.

We do take dreaming seriously, though, when the content of our dreams is particularly disturbing or guilt provoking. When this happens, we react by making the same mistake that we do with waking fantasies—that is, we blur the dividing line between fantasy and reality. This is particularly true when our dreams contain themes of a bizarre or antisocial sexual nature. Actually, bizarre sexual dreams are very common—dreams of incest, dreams of homosexuality, dreams about intercourse with a variety of sexually proscribed personages ranging from one's mother-in-law to the family dog. One type of dream that many men find extremely disturbing—that of having intercourse with a hermaphrodite, a woman who has a penis—is actually an extremely common motif found in the art and literature of many different cultures. We must learn not to expect dreams and fantasies to make sense in waking terms. Dreams and fantasies do not deal with permissible, commonplace subjects but instead with the socially unacceptable and illicit. If we hope to be comfortable with our sexuality, we must learn to accept the bizarre nature of our dreams and fantasies as being in the normal range.

The person who wishes to do so can go a step further than merely accepting his sexual dreams for what they are. He can learn to regulate and modify his dreams to some extent. Given the proper technique and a little practice, we can "program" our dreams, introduce themes and characters of our own choosing, and thus bring our dreams, along with our fantasies, within the province of our personal, imaginary Hollywood. The technique involved is to decide who and what you would like to dream about on a particular evening. As you fall asleep, keep that idea fixed in your mind. Chances are that the chosen material will appear in your dreams in some form that night or at a subsequent time. This is a technique I often use, combining travel and exotic sexual adventures as dream themes. The result may not be exactly what you ordered, but the fact that the technique can be used with some success shows that it is possible to modify something that is potentially distressing and remove its threatening aspects. It also shows that if we can separate our propensity to impose moral judgments from the enjoyment connected with our dream and fantasy activities, then our sexual dreams and fantasies can become a free and harmless source of entertainment and pleasure of unlimited variety.

Sexual fantasies differ from dreams in that they occur during waking life, when we have more conscious control of our minds and are better able to choose thoughts to give our attention to. Fantasies can serve as a bountiful source of pleasure and a convenient safety valve to draw off the accumulated pressures of our rational lives. If we keep in mind the distinction between fantasy and reality, between thought and act, then fantasy can be a way of allowing ourselves to indulge in those wishes and desires that are inappropriate or unacceptable to us and our society.

Two of the most common fantasies a man has when he sees a sexually attractive woman are to imagine what she would look like naked and what it would be like to have intercourse with her. Mentally undressing a woman and fantasizing intercourse with her substitutes for the actual behavior, which is socially inappropriate. Many men experience a conflict between their professed attitudes of respect for women and the content of their fantasies, but if the distinction between enjoying a fantasy about doing something and actually wanting to do it is kept firmly in mind, then the fantasy can be enjoyed without any accompanying guilt or anxiety. Having such fantasies does not mean that you are a male chauvinist who wants to rape every woman you see. A man can have an active fantasy life that contradicts every personal ethic he subscribes to without ever violating his beliefs in terms of actual behavior. By their nature, sexual fantasies involve socially unacceptable sexual activity. Almost no one fantasizes about having sex with his wife in his bedroom in the missionary position.

The opportunity to indulge in forbidden or impractical relationships is just one of the possible uses of sexual fantasy. It may also serve as a way of enhancing a relationship between two people who are in the process of becoming sexually involved. Sexual fantasies a man has about a woman he is dating may be a source of excitement and gratification for him and strengthen his interest in her. This is equally true whether the relationship is new or long-standing, whether it is intimate or merely at the flirtation stage. In fact, older married men could probably improve their sexual relationships with their wives by deliberately incorporating activities with their wives into their fantasies. For example, instead of your routine sexual scenario, fantasize about being sexual with your wife in a special, sexy outfit she wouldn't be comfortable wearing in real life, and imagine other couples looking on admiringly and commenting on your sexual technique. For men who desire greater novelty and spontaneity in marital sex, fantasizing about things they would really like may be the first step toward making them happen. In an intimate relationship, a great deal of pleasure may be derived from the sharing of sexual fantasies. For example, telling your wife about a fantasy of yours in which she comes into your office and seduces you can serve to heighten the erotic feelings between the two of you—though it is highly unlikely that either of you would want to act out this fantasy, unless you have a very private office.

A man's sexual fantasies about a woman can enhance their relationship in another, quite different way. Fantasy may serve as a rehearsal, a learning experience that can be particularly helpful for younger, less experienced males. Depending on his capacity for making his fantasies vivid and detailed, a man may rehearse an entire lovemaking scene again and again, revising and editing to his heart's content. As a result, the real-life event may go more smoothly when it actually occurs.

Fantasy can and is used as an accompaniment during sexual intercourse. In fact, as many as 75 percent of men fantasize during partner sex. The fantasies serve as a bridge to build greater sexual arousal. The experience of imagining having sex with another woman is a fairly common one, yet most people feel an acute sense of guilt at indulging in this type of fantasy. Such guilt is unnecessary, however, since changing a partner's identity in your imagination does not necessarily mean that you want to change it in real life. One of my students, a married man, liked to evoke a particular fantasy of multiple sex partners during intercourse with his wife. He would imagine that six women, one of whom was his wife, were making love to him. Two of them would be taking turns sucking his penis, another would be moving her finger in and out of his anus, a fourth would be massaging and sucking his nipples, a fifth presenting her vulva for him to explore with his tongue, and a sixth would be wildly rubbing her body against his. Other images would flit in and out of his mind, such as two of the women making love to one another while admiring his body, or three or four of them fighting to perform fellatio on him. Far from proving disturbing or guilt provoking, these fantasies served to heighten his arousal during marital sex.

As in the case of dreams, bizarre and antisocial themes are quite natural in sexual fantasies. Fantasy and reality are two distinct realms, and there is no need to feel guilty or disturbed about the content of any fantasy as long as it does not become obsessive or acted out in real life. It is natural, for example, to fantasize about having sex with women of a different race. Group sex, anal sex, forced sex, observing others having sex, and sadomasochistic experiences are common subjects of fantasies. Violent and aggressive sexual fantasies are quite normal. Homosexual fantasies are common, too, and do not mean that a man is a repressed homosexual. Homosexual fantasies are the fourth most common theme among heterosexual men and heterosexual fantasies are the third most common theme among homosexual men. Tom, another student of mine, reported that he occasionally enjoyed having a homosexual fantasy. While masturbating, he would imagine that there were two handsome and muscular men who were his sexual slaves. One would perform anal intercourse on him while the other blew him. Although he found the fantasy quite arousing, it was not something that he wanted to carry through to behavior. He accepted homosexuality as valid for gay people, but he was quite satisfied as a functioning heterosexual who had occasional homosexual fantasies.

SUMMING UP

Sexual fantasies, rather than being something to fear and avoid, can be a great source of pleasure for any person. No fantasy is "sick" or "immoral" as long as it remains a fantasy; in fact, bizarre and antisocial fantasies are very common. The danger is not in the fantasy itself but in the guilt that may accompany it, for it is guilt that can make us focus obsessively on one particular fantasy, thus limiting the variety of sexual stimuli we find arousing. My clinical experience has shown that the healthiest and most rewarding practice is to cultivate a number of different fantasies, to enjoy them all, and to feel guilty about none of them. In this way, fantasy can become a help to us rather than a threat. Fantasy can serve to amuse, to excite, to educate, and to refresh us. Fantasies serve as a mental bridge to increase involvement and arousal during partner sex. It can make the experience of being male and being sexual a richer and more rewarding one.

14
COMFORT AND PLEASURE WITH ORAL SEX

Consider the mouth. What a marvelously sensitive and expressive part of the body it is! Our mouths have a wonderful ability to receive and analyze sensations. Best of all, our mouths have an enormous capacity for experiencing pleasure. Think of the enjoyment of biting into a juicy steak or of downing a chilled beer on a sweltering day.

Like our mouths, our genitals are richly supplied with nerve endings and exquisitely receptive to pleasurable sensations. Isn't it natural and fitting then that, in seeking to experience and to impart sexual pleasure, we employ oral-genital stimulation? For our mouths and our sex organs, which have so much in common and so much to offer one another, can unite to produce a very special and intense pleasure.

We are accustomed to using our mouths, our lips, and our tongues, to kiss, suck, lick, nibble, and bite the lips, face, breasts, and other parts of our partner's body. Oral-genital stimulation is nothing more than a normal extension of this. It is a coming together of the two most sensitive pleasure-giving and pleasure-receiving areas of the body. This is equally true of fellatio, the oral stimulation of the penis, and cunnilingus, the oral stimulation of the vulva. Both are natural and healthy activities that are not only well within the normal range of sexual expression but also represent a comfortable, integrated attitude toward sexuality. Studies indicate that couples who enjoy oral sex rate their sexual lives more satisfying than couples who avoid oral sex because of discomfort, inhibition, or believing in the myth that it's a perverse type of sexual activity.

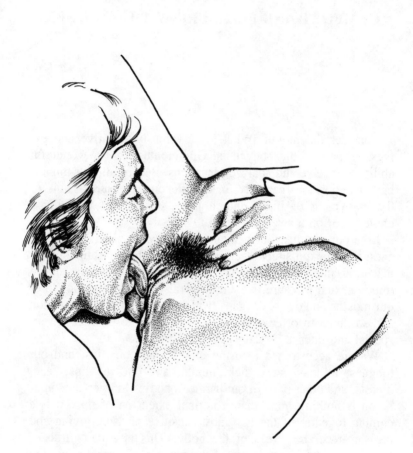

Oral sex. We often forget just how marvelously sensitive and expressive the mouth is.

MYTHS ABOUT ORAL SEX

Unfortunately, a whole complex of predjudices and misconceptions has grown up around the subject of oral-genital sex, causing many people to shy away from this method of sexual expression or, if they indulge in it, to feel anxious and guilty about their activity. Let us consider some of these negative attitudes toward oral-genital sex and try to understand and dispel the myths and inhibitions that prevent this form of sexuality from being more freely and comfortably practiced.

One of the major misconceptions about oral-genital sex is that it is unclean—that is, not sanitary. Americans in particular have a concern, practically an obsession, with oral cleanliness, which is reflected in the endless succession of ads for toothpaste, mouthwashes, and breath mints seen in magazines and on television. The genitals, on the other hand, are considered a "dirty" part of the body, not only because of the lingering puritanical attitudes toward sex but also because of the close connection between the sex organs and the organs of excretion. The male urethra serves as a channel not only for semen but for urine as well; and the female expels urine through the urethral meatus, located between the clitoris and the vagina. In contemplating the idea of orally stimulating the genitals of a partner, many people are dismayed by the prospect of taking into the mouth organs that have been contaminated by urine.

But such concerns are quite unfounded. If a person washes properly, then no remnant of urine will remain on the genitals. Many people prefer to wash their genitals before engaging in sexual activity, especially oral-genital sex. With ordinary hygiene, the sex organs can be as germ free and clean smelling as any other part of the body. In fact, the mouth usually contains a great many more germs than the penis or vulva. Sexual secretions—the male's semen and the lubricating fluids of the female—are antiseptic and perfectly harmless protein substances.

The factor most responsible for negative attitudes toward oral-genital sex is an ignorance of the structure and function of the genitals—your own and those of your partner. Mutual examination and self-examination of the genital area can be an enlightening and often liberating experience for a couple, and may serve to change their attitudes toward oral-genital sex.

One of my clients, a young, married law student who had

been very active sexually and was proud of his masculinity and sexual prowess, experienced such a psychological breakthrough. He very much enjoyed being fellated by his wife, but he was anxious and uncomfortable with the experience of cunnilingus and would usually avoid doing it even if she requested it. Not surprisingly, this created a sense of sexual imbalance and tension in the marital relationship. Originally, they had come to me for therapy to reduce their anxiety about childbirth, but as therapy progressed, the strife caused by his attitude toward oral-genital sex emerged as a significant problem. He claimed to be disgusted by the fact that the urethra was located in the vulva area. "Piss just doesn't turn me on," was the way he expressed it. At my suggestion, he agreed to make a thorough visual inspection of his wife's genitals. The experience was a turning point. He realized that while the urethra was indeed located in the vulva area, he could avoid it if he chose by concentrating on the clitoral shaft, inner lips, and the vagina. His anxiety was reduced considerably, and he was able to enjoy orally stimulating his wife. He found it particularly arousing if she fellated him at the same time.

This example shows not only the value of direct knowledge of sexual anatomy in overcoming hang-ups but also the importance of choice in oral-genital sex (or in any phase of sexuality). While therapy techniques such as the one described above can be helpful in changing our attitudes and behavior, we should not allow ourselves to be forced by outside pressure (including this book) into any sexual activity we feel uncomfortable about. Our sex lives should be motivated by genuine desire and the wish to experiment and increase our sources of pleasure, not by a sense of duty or in an effort to prove you are sexually liberated. You may decide that oral-genital sex is just not for you, but why not be adventurous enough to give it a fair chance?

Vaginal secretions have a definite flavor of their own—a salty, tangy, complex taste that is really not quite like anything else. Many men enjoy this taste and find it highly arousing. Others may not find it quite so appealing. While it is useless to try to persuade someone to like something he does not enjoy, it is nevertheless true that tastes may be acquired, particularly when the surrounding circumstances are positive.

The key to learning to enjoy the experience of cunnilingus is

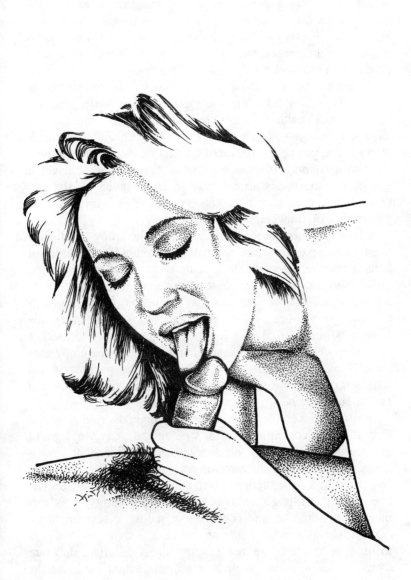

Oral-genital stimulation combines two of the most sensitive organs of the body.

to approach it in a gradual way. For example, a man might begin by caressing the woman's vulva with his lips closed. When he feels comfortable with this form of stimulation, he can progress to using his tongue and open mouth. There are several products on the market—flavored vaginal sprays—that are meant to appeal to women whose partners have ambivalent feelings about oral-genital sex. Some of these products are of dubious value from a health point of view, increasing the potential for vaginal infections, and should not be used. Others are hypoallergenic and can be used without a problem; the couple can pick out flavored sprays that appeal to the man. Other men feel it would be more honest to cultivate an appreciation for the real thing rather than to try to make it palatable with synthetic peppermint or strawberry flavoring.

A common misconception is that men who enjoy fellatio are latent homosexuals. While it is true that homosexual couples of both sexes use oral-genital techniques—often very skillfully and satisfyingly—it is not the technique employed that makes the act a homosexual one but the fact that the people involved are of the same sex. When two males erotically kiss each other, the activity is homosexual, but certainly kissing in and of itself is not a sign of latent homosexuality, and neither is the enjoyment of fellatio. Heterosexual men who report the greatest sexual satisfaction are more likely to enjoy both receiving fellatio and giving cunnilingus.

Oral-genital sex has been unjustly maligned in other ways. One frequent contention is that oral-genital sex is a sign of immaturity—the basis of this charge being the idea that heterosexual intercourse in the male-on-top position is the only truly "adult" form of sexuality. This, of course, is nonsense. The hallmark of fulfilling, healthy sexuality is the ability to experiment, communicate, and cooperate in mutual pleasuring techniques. Couples who limit their sexual activity to a single method or position are not proving their maturity; they are merely stuck in a rut. Their lack of imagination increases the possibility of becoming bored with sex altogether and developing a sexual dysfunction.

Oral-genital sex is an area a couple can explore to add variety to their sex life. In fact, surveys have indicated that those couples who practice oral-genital sex, rather than being characterized by immaturity, tend to be better educated and more sexually fulfilled. Approximately 85 percent of couples do experiment with oral-genital stimulation, and 50 percent use it with some frequency.

THE RELATIONSHIP BETWEEN ORAL SEX AND INTERCOURSE

Some men, who mistakenly think of oral-genital techniques as a substitute for intercourse, believe that the use of the mouth in sex is an indication of a lack of virility. This is particularly the case where cunnilingus is concerned. The assumption—based on a very narrow and rigid conception of sexuality—is that a man who orally stimulates a woman does so because he is incapable of satisfying her with his penis. Actually, a man who employs cunnilingus as part of his sexual repertoire is likely to be more relaxed and confident about his sexual ability. Consequently, he will probably be more competent, both in intercourse and in oral-genital techniques, than a man who limits his lovemaking to intercourse.

There is a fear, held by a surprising number of men, that a woman might become "addicted" to oral-genital sex and prefer it to intercourse. While it is true that many women find oral sex extremely pleasurable, since it provides more direct stimulation of the clitoral area, there is no evidence that they become indifferent to penile stimulation. On the contrary, couples who use oral-genital techniques are more likely to enjoy other methods of sexual activity, including, most definitely, intercourse. For intercourse and oral-genital sex are complementary, not either-or, activities. Most couples use fellatio and cunnilingus as pleasuring activities that generally lead to, and indeed whet the appetite for, intercourse.

Learning to see oral-genital sex as a natural, healthy, and permissible activity is an essential prerequisite to deriving the optimal degree of pleasure from it. We can then approach it in the mutually cooperative and guiding manner that characterizes the most satisfying sexual functioning.

Too often, men who desire oral-genital sex think of it as a forbidden pleasure that they must procure either by coercion or else outside the realm of their normal sexual relationship. The prevalence of this feeling is demonstrated by the fact that the majority of married men who go to prostitutes request fellatio rather than intercourse; they are unable to ask their wives to fellate them. These men seem to set up a strict dichotomy between the kind of sex allowed within marriage (only intercourse) and the sex they seek outside of marriage (where anything goes). There is no reason why such a dichotomy should exist. The mistaken belief that there are sexual activities that are not permissible for married couples has a great deal to do with perpetuating sexual dissatisfaction in marriage.

COMMUNICATING ABOUT ORAL SEX

Other men may try oral-genital sex with their wives but give it up when it does not go well at first. The man tells himself that since the woman does not seem particularly turned on by it, he is doing her a favor by not asking her to go through with it again. Such an attitude denies the woman's potential responsiveness to oral-genital sex as well as ignoring the complexity of fellatio and cunnilingus as sexual behaviors that require communication, comfort, guidance, and feedback that clearly cannot be achieved at the first opportunity. If couples reacted to their first intercourse experiences as they sometimes do to their first attempts at oral-genital sex, they would cease having intercourse altogether.

Oral-genital sex is something a man has a perfect right to request from his partner, just as she has a perfect right to request it from him. Not only can they feel comfortable asking for oral stimulation, but they ought to be able to guide one another in achieving the most satisfying kind of stimulation. A genuine give-and-take (using both verbal and nonverbal communication) between partners will enable them to find the best way of pleasuring one another. Too many men think of fellatio as a "symbolic" act rather than as a mutually pleasurable activity. They feel that just getting their partners to "go down on them" is really all they can expect. But there is much more to oral-genital sex than this.

The point is well illustrated by a couple who were clients of mine in sex therapy. The man had been pressing his wife for a long time to fellate him, but she could not get up the courage.

Finally, he convinced her to try it one evening when she was drunk. After overcoming her resistance this one time, she was able to repeat the act on a regular basis. Her husband, however, feeling that he had gotten what he wanted and had no right to request anything further from her, offered no feedback or guidance. She, meanwhile, had worked out her own method of fellating him, according to what seemed comfortable and arousing to her. Rather than taking the head of the penis into her mouth, she concentrated on sucking and stimulating the shaft. When I asked the man privately whether he was satisfied with the stimulation she had been giving he became very embarrassed. "Please don't tell my wife this," he said, "but actually I dislike the way she fellates me—it hurts!" He agreed to communicate his dissatisfaction to his wife, and eventually they did manage to work out a style of oral-genital stimulation that was satisfying to both of them.

There are several potential problems in oral-genital sex that are apt to arise chiefly because of a failure to communicate. For example, many women are reluctant to fellate their partners because of a fear of gagging on the penis. Rather than urging her to continue despite her discomfort or withdrawing a request out of a misplaced sense of compassion, the most appropriate response is to encourage her to experiment until she is able to fellate him with comfort. For example, she could try placing the penis to one side of her mouth rather than in the center, or she might try holding the shaft in her fingers as she takes it into her mouth. These techniques give the woman a greater sense of control and prevent the penis from going too deep so that the gag reflex is not triggered. A relaxed, nondemand atmosphere is best for reducing anxiety in both partners. Often the ability of the partners to laugh at the situation can be invaluable for relieving the awkwardness of the occasion. After all, sex—of whatever variety—is supposed to be fun!

Another problem that may arise is the woman's discomfort over the man's ejaculating in her mouth or her lack of desire to swallow the man's semen once he ejaculates, and the man's subsequent feeling that by rejecting his semen she is rejecting him. Here, again, we encounter a too-rigid approach to oral-genital sex and a failure of the partners to honestly and emphatically communicate their feelings. The man should realize that the woman's allowing him to ejaculate in her mouth or swallowing his semen is not the chief factor in the pleasure he receives from fellatio. Our main concern in sex should be pleasure, not symbolism. Besides, the woman's willingness or unwillingness relates to what is comfortable and pleasurable for her, not to any personal acceptance or rejection of her partner. There is no reason to expect fellatio to follow some set format, ending with ejaculation. Rather, whether it should be used simply as a pleasuring technique or can continue until the man reaches orgasm is a question that can be decided according to what is pleasurable and acceptable to both partners.

Of course, understanding and communicating are just as important for successful cunnilingus. Frequently, men who have not taken the trouble to examine their partner's anatomy or who have not received adequate guidance from her may use oral stimulation in ways that are ineffective. Two distinct problems arise here. On the one hand, the man might be concentrating his attention on the vagina or the outer lips, where the concentration of nerve endings is rather sparse, and thus be producing a minimum of pleasurable sensations. Or he might be stimulating the clitoris in a way that is too direct or rough and thereby cause more pain than pleasure.

The clitoris is an extremely sensitive organ, particularly at the tip or glans. Most women prefer indirect stimulation of the clitoris around the clitoral shaft rather than a direct focus on the glans. Different women respond to different types of oral stimulation. Some like slow, rhythmic stroking, while others prefer a rapid, focused movement. Still others like the man to run his tongue over the clitoris and then suck on the clitoral shaft and labia minora area. Many women find they are extremely responsive to oral stimulation, but only when they are already feeling some arousal. Doing cunnilingus when the woman is minimally aroused is usually counterproductive. Discuss with your partner the kind of stimulation she prefers and then follow her guidance. In any case, the ideal situation for sexual functioning is one in which this information can be imparted frankly and openly, in which it is recognized that each partner has the right—in fact, the responsibility—to request stimulation that is most effective for him or her. Sexual requests are best when they are clear and direct, and are not demands.

GETTING INTO ORAL SEX

For the couple wishing to improve their comfort and pleasure with oral-genital sex, the best approach to follow is a gradual one. Begin with manual stimulation of the genitals, with one partner taking the role of giver and the other that of recipient. Begin slowly to use oral stimulation, concentrating at first on the insides of the thighs and the area surrounding the genitals. Over the course of several sessions, work up gradually to direct oral stimulation of the genitals, experimenting with different types of movements such as licking, sucking, kissing, and a darting movement of the tongue. Keep the lines of communication open about your comfort and pleasure level; each partner can feel free to say what he or she likes and doesn't like. Once you have begun to feel comfortable with oral-genital sex, there is no end to the variations you can improvise. Many couples find mutual, simultaneous oral stimulation—the famous "69" position—to be extremely satisfying. Others find they are not comfortable receiving and giving stimulation at the same time and prefer to take turns being giver or recipient. Some people like oral sex best in the position where one is standing and the other is kneeling, other couples enjoy it best when one is lying down and the other is above. Some enjoy being passive while receiving oral sex, with the giver doing the movement, and others find it much more arousing to move when being stimulated.

Remember that the reason for engaging in oral-genital sex should be to enhance your pleasure, not to prove anything to yourself or anyone else. We should be wary of the new sexual conformism in which people feel pressured to show that they are free of sexual inhibitions by demonstrating their readiness to engage in every possible form of sexual behavior.

A particular sexual technique becomes the "in" thing, and people who like to think of themselves as being sexually liberated feel that they must try it and like it or else jeopardize their self-image. The latest of these sex fashions are analingus, the oral stimulation of the anus, and oral stimulation of the testicles, including taking the whole testicle into the mouth. There is nothing abnormal or "bad" about these particular techniques as long as proper hygiene is utilized and care is taken not to hurt the partner. What would be unfortunate, though, would be to do these things simply because you feel it is expected of you or out of a fear of being thought inhibited or unsophisticated.

Whether the sexual experience is analingus, group sex, bondage and discipline, swinging, or watching hard-core pornographic films in your bedroom, the same basic guideline applies. As long as a particular sexual activity is not forced, does not involve children, is not carried out in public, and is not compulsive or clearly destructive, it falls within the range of normal sexual variation. However, if you feel pressured to engage in certain acts to prove that you are liberated, you are no longer expressing your sexuality in your own best interest or to heighten intimacy in your relationship. The focus of sexuality is pleasure, not performing according to a certain standard—whatever that standard may be.

CLOSING THOUGHTS

I want to emphasize once again that the key to effective, satisfying oral-genital sex is gentleness, comfort, and communication. If you approach it in this way, you will soon find that it ceases to be a "heavy scene," potentially threatening and frustrating to both partners, and becomes a positive and healthy part of sexuality that enlarges the range of techniques you can use to express your love and passion for one another.

15
SEX AND THE AGING MALE

How difficult is it for you to picture your parents making love? What about your grandparents? How would you feel about seeing a picture of a nude seventy-year-old woman as the centerfold of *Playboy* or *Penthouse*? Or how about a nude man in his seventies as the centerfold of *Playgirl*? Are you turned off by these images? If you are, it is because you share the dominant tendency in our society to deny sexuality to older people. Where sex is concerned, you are a youth chauvinist.

Our culture considers itself to be sexually liberated, but the changes it advocates in sexual attitudes do not extend to all ages. Yes, sex has become freer, more open, but only for that segment of the population between adolescence and the middle years of adulthood. For those above or below these chronological boundaries, sexuality is still not supposed to exist. It is commonly assumed that neither children nor old people are capable of sexual feelings or entitled to any sort of sexual gratification. Children are expected to be innocent, pure, unaffected by sex. This may partially explain why many adults become so upset when children engage in self-stimulation or play sexual games such as "doctor" and "house." At the other end of the age scale, older people are considered to be "over the hill" sexually and are expected to lapse uncomplainingly into a peaceful, nonerotic state, free of all sexual thoughts, desire, and arousal.

In fact, we are sexual people from the day we are born to the day we die. Infants are capable of becoming sexually aroused and having erections. Men and women in their sixties, seventies, eighties, and beyond can and do have sexual desire, experience sexual excitement, are able to have intercourse, and can be orgasmic. In the chapter "Sex, Your Children, and You," we saw how important it is for parents to acknowledge the sexuality of their children, to allow them to explore and enjoy their bodies, and to provide them with a positive, unambiguous sex education. Here we will take a look at the role of sex in the life of the older man (and woman). What we will see is that, while a man's sexual responses change as he grows older, the aging man in good health is still quite capable of effective sexual functioning, of being an involved sex partner, and of being able to enjoy a variety of sexual activities, including intercourse. As a man grows older, he will find that sex is different from his younger days, but not necessarily less enjoyable. Older men might not be high-frequency sexual athletes, but they can be better sexual lovers.

THE NEGATIVE INFLUENCE OF OUR ATTITUDES

But if the older man is still capable of functioning sexually, why is it that so many men give up on sex as they enter their fifties and sixties? The answer is negative cultural conditioning. Our society simply has not included sexuality as part of the "role" elderly people are supposed to assume. This is not true of some other cultures, where it is considered quite natural for older people to show an open interest in sexuality and to lead active and fulfilling sex lives. Yet our society has long associated sexuality primarily with adolescents and young adults and tends to see sexual enjoyment as inappropriate for anyone beyond the childbearing years. Only rarely is the sexual activity of older persons presented in a sensitive, accepting manner by the media. More often, older men who openly express interest in sex are assumed to be "dirty old men" or even "perverts." Faced with such opposition, it is understandable that a large number of older men simply give up and content themselves with being nonsexual for the remainder of their lives. When couples stop having sex, in 95 percent of the cases, it is the man's decision.

Unfortunately, physicians, the very people older men rely on for information about aging, sometimes share the false idea that sex probably will end in the sixties. But after all, they are only reflecting our society's preconceptions. Many older doctors were trained when there were no sexuality courses in medical schools, and thus they may be unfamiliar with recent scientific findings about sex and aging. It is not uncommon to find older men discouraged from pursuing an active sex life or being old that they must accept the loss of sexual desire and functioning as a part of the aging process. Some doctors, along with many laymen, seem to think that sexual dysfunction is a natural part of the aging process. But this is simply not true.

Feeling unsure about their right to sexual feelings, many older people block sexual thoughts from their minds because they feel that such ideas are wrong or unnatural. As a result of such self-imposed mental censorship, many older men repress sexual desire and feelings. Others, while remaining in touch with their sexual feelings, may become convinced that they are no longer capable of acting upon them. If a man believes or fears that he cannot get an erection, his attitudes may well prevent him from getting one. This experience of erectile dysfunction will then serve to reinforce his original belief that he is no longer a sexual person, and, as a result, he will eventually resign himself to a life without sexual activity.

NORMAL CHANGES WITH AGING

But there is no real reason why an older man should have to make such a sacrifice. Sexual functioning does not cease naturally with aging. Studies show that men, no matter what their age and whether or not they are active sexually, continue to have regular erections during sleep. If a man can get an erection in his sleep, he should also be able to get one with a partner. If he can get an erection with a partner, he should be able to have and enjoy sexual activity, including, but not limited to, intercourse. In fact, there is no more reason for a man to lose his ability to have sex than for him to lose the ability to perform any other natural physical function. A man of seventy may not be able to run as fast as he could when he was twenty, but if he has kept himself in good condition he will be able to take a brisk walk. Similarly, a man who has remained sexually active into old age will not respond as rapidly to sexual stimulation or ejaculate as frequently, but he will still be able to enjoy sex on a regular basis. The important thing is for a man to realize that sexual pleasure is something he can and should have as he grows older. Sexuality is a part of life. As long as he is alive, a man has a right to be sexual and to find pleasure in sexual expression.

One major reason why many older men become discouraged with sex is that they are not well prepared for the changes in sexual response that gradually occur as a result of aging. If he doesn't understand them, an aging man is liable to misinterpret these changes as a sign that he is losing his sexual ability. Consequently, he may become uneasy about his capacity to satisfy his partner and either avoid sex altogether or become so anxious about performing well that sex is no longer enjoyable for him. But there is no reason why this should happen. If men are aware of what to expect in gradually changing sexual functioning (and share this knowledge with their partners), they should be able to derive as much enjoyment from sex as ever—in some ways, even more.

When he was in his teens and twenties, the man could get "automatic" erections and function autonomously (i.e., he needed nothing from the woman in order to experience desire, achieve erection, and reach orgasm). However, for most men in their forties, and almost all men by their sixties, sex is a sharing, cooperative activity with the woman. Actually, all the lessons on respectful, cooperative male-female relationships, the enjoyment of nondemand pleasuring, and the need for multiple stimulation come to fruition with the aging process. The man who is aware of and accepting of these concepts before age sixty is in an excellent position to make a positive transition to sex and aging.

One change that commonly occurs with aging is a decrease in the need and desire for ejaculation. This, like most sexual changes, usually begins between the ages of fifty and sixty, although there is a great deal of variation from one individual to another. Older men often find that they do not desire to ejaculate each time they have intercourse, even though they may be aroused and enjoy the sexual experience. If a man does not feel the need on a particular occasion, he should not try to force the ejaculation but rather just enjoy the sensations of intercourse. Vasocongestion of the testicles during sexual arousal is not as pronounced in older men, so there will not be a problem with "blue balls" as a result of not ejaculating.

This decrease in the urge for ejaculation is a natural change and is not to be confused with ejaculatory inhibition. The aging man should accept this change and not try to force himself to ejaculate when he has no genuine need or desire. When ejaculation does occur, there are some differences. The older man will find that his ejaculation might last a shorter time than before, that his penis might contract fewer times, that semen might come out less forcefully, and that less semen might be ejaculated. Instead of ejaculation being a two-step process, consisting of the point of ejaculatory inevitability followed by the ejaculation itself, it will occur as a single-stage process—that is, he will not experience the feeling of inevitability before ejaculating. Thus, sex becomes less ejaculation oriented but not necessarily less pleasure oriented.

Some men report they actually experience an orgasm without ejaculating. Other men report that even though they did not have an orgasm or ejaculate they enjoyed the sexual experience; and some even report experiencing an intensity of pleasure equivalent to orgasm.

Another difference is that once an older man has ejaculated, he finds that his penis becomes flaccid much faster than it did in earlier years. This causes the man to fear he is losing his sexual powers and that he may not be able to achieve an erection next time. This fear may be connected with the fact that the older man experiences a longer refractory period. That is, following ejaculation, he will not be able to achieve another erection for a period varying from several hours to a full day, while as a young man he might have been able to get a second erection in an hour or less. Such anxiety is unjustified, however. The fact that a man's sexual responses are slowing down doesn't mean that they are about to stop altogether. If he is willing to accept the new sexual pace that comes with aging, he will find that sex can be satifying. The adage that as one ages he is less of a sexual athlete, but more a sensuous lover, is a good one.

One definite advantage of the less urgent need to ejaculate is that he far exceeds the younger man in ejaculatory control. This greater control can be utilized so that he and his partner can enjoy intercourse to the fullest. As sex becomes less ejaculation oriented, the older man is able to relax and become receptive to the myriad, subtle, whole-body sensations of lovemaking. In the sense that his ability to both give and receive pleasure is increased, a man becomes a better lover as he grows older.

Along with the lessened need for ejaculation, the whole process of sexual arousal tends to be slower as a man ages. For example, while a younger man may require only seconds of stimulation before getting an erection, an older man may need several minutes or more. In addition, older men need more direct stimulation of the penis to become fully aroused. A young man may get an erection just from thinking about sex, or from seeing his partner's nude body. With older men it is necessary for the partner to use the stroking or rubbing stimulation the man finds most arousing. Once achieved, the erection of an older man is often not as full as in earlier days, but as long as it is firm enough to allow penetration this need not be a source of concern. Even if the penis is not completely erect, the man's partner can help guide it into her vagina, and after several thrusts the strength of the erection will increase.

FEMALE CHANGES

A woman's sexual responses change as she grows older, just as a man's do. For women, however, menopause (which is typically a two-year process occurring between ages forty-five and fifty-five) serves as a clear milestone of physical change, whereas changes in a man's body are more gradual and less obvious. In addition to the cessation of menstruation, the aging woman finds that her vagina becomes somewhat smaller in size and that the vaginal walls become thinner and less elastic; the breasts and the clitoris might also decrease in size. Despite these changes, a woman's body continues to be responsive to sexual stimulation. Like her male counterpart, the aging woman's response pattern is much the same as it was when she was younger, but somewhat slower. Actually, changes in female sexual response are less than in males.

For instance, it will take the older woman longer to become lubricated when she becomes sexually excited, and the amount of lubrication will not be as great as when she was younger. Because of this, many older couples find it helpful to use a sterile lubricating jelly such as K-Y Jelly or a nonallergenic lotion, both available without a prescription. Saliva can also serve as an excellent and perfectly safe lubricant. One common fear that aging couples have is that menopause will put an end to the woman's sexual desire. Hysterectomy (the surgical removal of the uterus) is also frequently thought of as being the death knell of a woman's sexuality. Neither of these beliefs is valid. In fact, a woman may feel freer and more sexual after she has lost her ability to reproduce, since she no longer has to worry about the danger of an unwanted pregnancy. The more the woman and man know about menopause and female aging the less likely it is that these things will have any negative effects on sexual expression.

POSITIVE ELEMENTS OF THE AGING PROCESS

It is apparent that aging brings with it certain definite changes in the sexual functioning of both men and women. These changes, however, are not indications that a person's sex life is over, but rather that it is entering a new phase, taking on a new style. Sex between older people tends to be slower, gentler, and more interactive than in earlier years. An older man can focus on experiencing and giving pleasure rather than on turning in a good performance. He needs to be able to communicate and feel comfortable requesting specific types of stimulation, especially direct penile stimulation.

It helps if he can learn to appreciate other aspects of sex besides intercourse and orgasm—open himself to the limitless possibilities of increased sensual awareness and pleasuring. In short, an older man must learn and utilize the guidelines that have been presented throughout this book if he is to continue leading an active sex life. He must learn, if he has not already done so, to be a lover rather than a stud. As he grows older, the changes in his body will help him make this adjustment, provided he accepts them. But if he fights the course of nature, he is bound to lose. Being a sexual man of seventy is different from being a sexual man of twenty. But the essence of sexuality— pleasure and sharing—is still central.

Aging itself is not an illness, but rather a natural physiological process. The more a man takes care of himself, eats well, maintains a regular sleep pattern, exercises regularly, does not smoke and if he drinks does so in moderation, and stays in good general health, the better his body will adjust to aging and the better his sexual functioning will be. One mistake that aging men make is to assume that frequent sexual contacts will wear them out or use up their sexual abilities. Older men who find that they are unable to get an erection or ejaculate on a particular occasion decide to avoid sex for a month or two and give themselves a rest. This is definitely the wrong approach. You do not need a rest from sex. What you do need is to have sex on a regular basis. The idea that a man only has a certain number of ejaculations and that when they are used up his sex life is over is totally false. In fact, the more regular his sexual expression, the easier it is to continue functioning sexually. A popular phrase is "Use it or lose it." A regular rhythm of sexual expression facilitates sexual functioning in the man and woman. By continuing to be affectionate and sensual in his relationship, by having intercourse and ejaculating regularly, an older man maintains the self-confidence he needs to lead an active sex life.

SEXUALITY AND ILLNESS

Of course, not all older men are in good physical health, and it is well known that certain diseases (for instance, cancer and kidney dysfunction) can interfere with satisfactory sexual functioning. In fact, almost any kind of illness will inhibit sexual activity, but it does not have to end it. Too often, men who have had prostate surgery, a heart attack, a stroke, lung disease, diabetes, and other illnesses assume that they can no longer be sexually active. If you do have an illness, you should try to gain as full an understanding of it as possible, including its effect on your sexuality. Consult your physician, accompanied by your wife if possible, and explain that sex is an important part of your life together and that you would like to know what changes you will have to make in your sexual activities, if any. Remember, however, that some physicians have little training in sexuality and may not be very comfortable or competent discussing your sexual problems.

If you are not satisfied with the advice that your general physician gives you, the next step would be to consult a physician with a subspecialty in sexual medicine. He should be able to explain clearly how your sexual functioning may be affected by your illness or by any medication you may be taking. If you do have an illness that places limitations on your sex life, then it is best for you to discuss these problems openly with your partner and physician. You and your partner need to vent your feelings and to communicate about your sexual relationship. Even in cases where intercourse may be very limited or impossible (as in some forms of chronic diabetes) there are other ways in which a couple can continue to provide pleasurable, sensual, and sexual experiences for each other, including oral and manual stimulation, hugging, massage, and so forth.

While a disease might limit a man's ability to have erections, his ability to have orgasms usually remains unimpaired. Thus, it can be quite pleasurable for him to continue sensual and sexual interactions. Too many couples are willing to give up sex entirely when illness or some other physical incapacity strikes. As a culture, we are too used to thinking of sex as something just for the young, the strong, and the healthy. In fact, sexual pleasure is one of the basic constants of life. It is available to both the young and the old, the healthy and the not so healthy. A person need not give up on sex or try to convince someone else that his or her sexual days are over. Sexuality, physical affection, intimacy, and communication help to make life enjoyable. A person is entitled to be sexual, whatever his age or physical condition.

In a small number of men between the ages of fifty-five and sixty-five, a decrease in testosterone level occurs that affects their ability to function sexually. These men can derive a great deal of benefit from consulting a physician and receiving testosterone replacement therapy. This is similar to the hormone replacement therapy often prescribed for women when they go through menopause.

Older couples who have sexual dysfunction problems use their age as an excuse to avoid seeking treatment. This is an unjustified fear since therapists report a success rate of about 70 percent with couples in their fifties, sixties, and seventies. Success in sex therapy depends on the couple's commitment to each other and their desire to enjoy satisfactory sexual functioning, not on how old they are.

Karl and Trudy

Karl and Trudy, for example, were in their mid-seventies when they came to me for sex therapy. Karl had owned a small chemical plant and had been actively involved in running the business until just a few years before. He decided that he wanted to spend the rest of his life enjoying hobbies and activities that he never had time for while he was working. So, he sold the business and retired. The transition from active businessman to perpetual vacationer was a difficult one for Karl. This is not unusual—the two most common problems for retired males are depression and alcoholism (both of which have clear negative effects on sexual functioning). The lack of self-respect that he began to feel manifested itself as an erection problem. Karl and Trudy had resigned themselves to a life without sexual interaction until Trudy confided the problem to their minister and he suggested that they consult a sex therapist. Once they accepted the idea that it was not normal for sexual functioning to stop in old age, Karl and Trudy began to make rapid progress. We used the same nondemand pleasuring exercises employed by younger couples, and their response was very positive. After a few sessions they were making love more frequently and with more pleasure than they had for the past twenty years. Also, Karl made changes in how he structured his time, and he made a more positive adjustment to retirement, which enhanced his psychological and sexual well-being.

OLDER, SINGLE MALES

So far, we have been dealing only with the older married man. What about the man who is either widowed or divorced? While many of these men may find other partners, a good number face the problem of feeling sexual urges yet not having a partner to interact with sexually. One valid outlet is masturbation. Our culture tends to view masturbation as appropriate mainly for boys and young men. However, masturbation can be an important and healthy means of sexual expression for the older man as well. And no one should feel guilty about using masturbation as a sexual outlet. Many older men (including well-functioning married men) do, in fact, masturbate, and this activity is just as normal for them as it is for any young man.

It is also quite common for older single men to remarry. Because women, on the average, have an eight-years-greater life expectancy than men, the number of women in proportion to men increases steadily with age. Therefore, an older man who wishes to remarry generally finds no shortage of available partners. Those who do remarry, however, often make the mistake of seeing their second marriage as a replacement for the first one. In establishing a new emotional and sexual relationship, it is important to view it as something new and unique, rather than compare it with the first marriage. Since it is a new relationship, you will need to be aware of the preferences and feelings of your new partner and be able to communicate your own needs and desires. Don't assume that the things that worked in the last relationship will work in this one. You will need to explore, be spontaneous, and communicate so that you can establish a satisfying emotional and sexual relationship.

CLOSING THOUGHTS

The attempt to set an age limit to sexuality is both unrealistic and unjust. We never outgrow sex, nor does a healthy man or woman ever entirely lose his or her desire and ability to function sexually. Even where physical disability is present, the need for sensual and sexual expression remains, and this need can be acknowledged and acted upon. The couple who remains together and is able to function sexually in old age is extremely fortunate. They should not feel self-conscious about their continuing desire for each other but rather feel proud of keeping their relationship so vital and take advantage of it to the fullest. If they understand and accept the unique characteristics of sex in the later years, they may be surprised to find their sexual relationship becoming more sensitive, sharing, tender, and enjoyable than it was in their earlier years.

16
REGAINING SEXUAL DESIRE

Sexual desire problems are "in" for the 1980s. The most important sex therapy book for professionals in this decade is about assessment and treatment of inhibited sexual desire. But isn't sexual desire a problem solely for women? In this macho culture of ours, where a "real man" wants to have sex with any woman, anytime, and in any situation, can there be any problem with male desire? The traditional view is that a man, especially a young man, is controlled by his rock-hard penis: "A hard cock has no conscience."

The reality is that problems of inhibited sexual desire occur on occasion for almost every man. For about ten to fifteen percent of men it is a chronic problem that becomes more severe over time. In our culture, it's easier to admit to a performance dysfunction (rapid ejaculation, erectile dysfunction, ejaculatory inhibition) than to a lack of sexual desire. Strong sexual desire is viewed as a natural characteristic of male sexuality and as a measure of masculinity. The sense of embarrassment over having a desire problem is so great for males that they resist entering into psychotherapy or sex therapy. If he is coerced into therapy with his partner, his goal is to minimize the problem and get out of therapy as quickly as possible.

Most men blame desire problems on some outside source (their job, their spouse's weight, lack of time, sex's becoming routine, etc.) and believe they need a "magic pill" or an outside source (a twenty-year-old sexy woman) to regain desire. It's as if desire isn't a personal part of the man but is controlled from external sources or the cultural stereotype of masculinity.

INHIBITIONS THAT BLOCK SEXUAL DESIRE

Psychologically, the key element in sexual desire is positive anticipation. Positive anticipation is an internal characteristic based on the man's attitudes and expectations regarding his sexuality and his partner. Although desire is certainly influenced by physiological factors (especially being in good health and the male hormone, testosterone), for most men that is not the primary problematic factor. There are medical factors that can lower sexual desire, such as illness, side effects of medication, drug or alcohol abuse, hormonal imbalance, fatigue or stress, and poor health habits. These can be evaluated in a general medical exam by your internist or family practice physician. The man hopes the problem is a medical one that he can take a pill for so it will magically disappear. However, when there is no medical malfunction (which is true for the great majority of males), he needs to examine psychological, relational, and situational causes.

The best way to understand the problem is by becoming aware of "inhibitions" that block positive anticipation, thus the professional term *inhibited sexual desire*. Sex therapists define primary inhibited sexual desire as the man never having had positive anticipation about sex with a partner. This is rare among men, although it is more common among women since our culture gives less permission for women to anticipate and express their sexuality. Common causes for primary inhibited sexual desire among men are a fixation on a masturbatory technique or fantasy (usually a fetish arousal pattern), trauma caused by child sex abuse or incest, conflict regarding sexual orientation, or negative attitudes toward sex, often governed by rigid religious beliefs or a strong antisex family environment.

Far more common is secondary inhibited sexual desire which affects up to 15 percent of men, and perhaps up to 33 percent of men over fifty. In fact, one of the most interesting statistics is that when older couples stop having sex, in over ninety percent of the cases it is the man's decision to stop being sexual. This decision is conveyed indirectly and nonverbally.

The most common cause for secondary inhibited sexual desire is an existing sexual dysfunction. The man's sexual dysfunction sets the stage for a pattern of negative anticipation, aversive sexual experience, followed by increasingly long periods of sexual avoidance. As the man's sense of frustration and failure increases, his sexual anticipation and desire decreases, and he actively avoids any sexual thoughts or interactions.

A second major cause of inhibited sexual desire is the man who used to function "automatically" (needing nothing from his partner) finds that as he ages, or as he lets sex get into a routine and stagnant scenario, automatic functioning is no longer possible. Rather than communicating with his partner and developing a more cooperative, giving sexual relationship, he chooses to withdraw and avoid, hoping "horniness" will develop from deprivation. This is a self-defeating strategy since a key element in sexual desire is a regular rhythm of sexual expression. For example, testosterone increases after orgasm. The pattern of avoidance leads to increased sexual avoidance and decreased sexual desire. Thus, the man sets himself (and his relationship) on a path of much reduced sexual expression.

A third cause is negative emotional responses, especially anxiety, depression, or anger. Sexuality is associated with positive emotions and motivations; negative emotions can and do inhibit desire. The negative emotions, both sexual and nonsexual, need to be dealt with directly so they don't control sexual expression. Much of sex therapy focuses on reducing sexual anxiety and replacing it with greater sexual comfort. Sexual anxiety is the negative emotion easiest to treat. Lowered sexual desire is one of the clinical signs of depression. Men tend to deny feeling depressed and go on with their routines at work and home, but to do so with minimal involvement and pleasure. Males prefer antidepressant medication as their way to deal with depression rather than examining and changing the psychological, relational, and situational factors that cause and maintain their depression (which as a psychologist I would strongly advise the man to do). Antidepresssant drugs actually have a negative effect on sexual functioning, but with the lifting of the depression, the net sexual effect is usually positive. Sexual desire does not automatically return with the lifting of the man's depressed mood, but the man can then reinvolve himself in fantasy, anticipation, and sexual touching with his partner. Anger is the most difficult emotion to deal with because males will often stubbornly hang on to their anger. Being "right" and winning the angry power struggle becomes more important than resuming the sexual relationship. Often the anger is about non-sexual issues, but it poisons the sexual relationship. The longer the anger is held and the more it is expressed through verbal and/or physical violence, the more detrimental it is to sexual desire (this is equally true for the female). The man and couple need to express the angry feelings in nondestructive ways, explore the hurt that is often the basis of the anger, problem-solve to resolve the conflicts and reach agreements both people can live with.

Alcohol and drug abuse (especially cocaine and barbiturates) have long-term negative effects on sexual desire. This is partic-ularly paradoxical, since reducing sexual inhibitions was one of the supposed functions of alcohol. Initially, cocaine had been touted as the "perfect aphrodiasiac." In truth, drug and alcohol abuse have a number of physical and psychological effects that inhibit sexual desire. Desire is not going to return until the substance abuse is successfully treated.

Relationship problems are another major cause of inhibited sexual desire. Men have a strong tendency to take their marriage for granted and allow it to become dull and routine. Relation-ships need attention to thrive. It's easy to fall into the trap of becoming frustrated with the relationship, and instead of its being a growth-enhancing, positive influence the marriage de-generates into a bitter standoff. The marital bond of respect, trust, and intimacy needs to be revitalized to regain sexual desire.

There are a number of other causes of inhibited sexual desire, including acute or chronic illness, sexual phobias or aversions, fear of pregnancy, negative attitudes toward sexuality, difficulty with children or jobs, lack of time with partner, and so on. The man and the couple need to be honest in identifying the factors that block sexual desire and instituting a plan for change. Inhib-ited sexual desire is a problem that usually requires professional therapy.

Jonathan

Regaining sexual desire is a function of the man's increasing his awareness, assuming greater responsibility for his sexuality, and working cooperatively with his partner to develop a sexual style that is functional and satisying for them. Jonathan presents a good illustration of this complex, yet achievable process. Jonathan is a forty-three-year-old consulting engineer who had allowed sexuality to slip away from him in the past five years. Jonathan had been having difficulty maintaining an erection during intercourse. On some occasions he experienced ejaculatory inhibition and on other occasions rapid ejaculation. Rather than discussing this with his wife and working with her to develop a more arousing and fulfilling sexual scenario, he became more distant from her emotionally and sexually.

The sexual difficulties left him vulnerable to an affair with his partner's secretary. The affair began as a very exciting and sexually fulfilling one. The sexual novelty and illicitness along with the psychological charge from feeling desired and attractive carried Jonathan for three months. However, things started collapsing like a house of cards. His partner was infuriated with Jonathan since the secretary had previously been doing marginal work and now her work was clearly unsatisfactory. Jonathan's own work was suffering, and clients were complaining to other partners. The affair became a major source of office gossip, and colleagues were saying very unkind things behind his back. Finally, someone from the office made an anonymous phone call to his wife, who then confronted Jonathan. She felt hurt, confusion, and anger. At first Jonathan tried to deny everything, which only made things worse. The breakup of the affair extended over six months (affairs are much easier to get into than out of), and by the end Jonathan was experiencing sexual dysfunction both in his marriage and in the affair. As the debris settled, he withdrew emotionally and sexually. Jonathan decided he would stay away from sex since it had caused so much pain and embarrassment in his life. For the next two years, his only sexual outlet was masturbation, which he put down as an adolescent behavior.

Jonathan was forced into therapy by his frustrated and angry wife, who wanted to deal with the past affair and the lack of sex in their relationship. To say that he was a reluctant client is a gross understatement; he saw nothing in therapy for him except further embarrassment and failure. Negative motivation seldom promotes positive behavior, so the first therapeutic task was to identify goals for him. Jonathan was encouraged to view his masturbation differently—the fact that he felt desire, got aroused, had an erection, and enjoyed orgasm reassured him that everything was intact physiologically and that sex could be a source of pleasure and satisfaction. The next step was attitudinal. He needed to view his wife as his sexual friend rather than his harshest sexual critic. Jonathan and his wife began a series of sexual exercises to rebuild a sense of comfort, attraction, and trust in the relationship. The psychological issues of anger and resentment were dealt with in the couple's therapy sessions. Jonathan came to enjoy the nondemand, nongoal-oriented pleasuring sessions as adding a new dimension to his life and revitalizing his marital relationship. Rather than sex being a drain on his self-esteem, it began to be an energizing force, a way of sharing pleasure, reducing frustration, and building intimacy.

REGAINING SEXUAL DESIRE

In regaining sexual desire and building positive anticipation about sexuality, there are factors the man needs to be aware of and responsible for. The first is an increased commitment to rebuilding his sexual self-esteem and honestly assessing (rather than avoiding, denying, or minimizing) the elements that are blocking his sexual desire. He can do this on his own, with a therapist, or with his partner, but he needs to make a commitment to honestly identifying the inhibitions and developing a plan for change. Self-exploration/masturbation exercises accompanied by experimentation with sexual fantasies are the most powerful individual interventions. This method allows the man to regain his confidence in a situation where he exerts control. In addition, it permits him to get back in touch with the kinds of stimulation that are turn-ons and build anticipation about being sexual. Additional individual interventions focus on making positive changes in his self-esteem and body image. These can include stopping smoking or drinking, beginning a weight-reduction or exercise program, practicing better personal hygiene, dressing in a more attractive manner, and so forth.

Another individual technique is to think out, talk out, write out, or fantasize about the sexual scenario that would be most desirable for you. Design a scenario that would lead to positive sexual anticipation. What would the foreplay/pleasuring be like? How would intercourse be initiated, what position would you enjoy most, what kind of thrusting and other stimulation would you use? How would the afterplay/afterglow sequence be played out? What are the elements in a sexual experience with your partner that would enhance your sense of emotional and sexual satisfaction?

COUPLE ISSUES IN INHIBITED SEXUAL DESIRE

More than any other sexual difficulty, inhibited sexual desire involves the couple's relationship. The famous story in sex therapy is the woman who came to a sex therapy clinic with her second husband. The problem was sexual desire. The therapist recalled that the woman had been at the clinic five years before with her first husband, when the problem had been that he wanted to be sexual twice a day and she wanted to be sexual twice a week. With her second husband, she still wanted to be sexual twice a week, but he only desired to be sexual once a month. Sexual desire problems are best conceptualized as a discrepancy in expectations. There is not a "right" or "normal" number of times to have intercourse. Couples need to develop their own style of being sexual—there is not "one right" style or right frequency. While the suggested exercises provide guidelines to experiment with, I encourage each couple to do what is comfortable for them.

The chief cause of inhibited sexual desire is taking the relationship for granted. If we put as little thought and energy into our businesses as we do into our marriages, there would be a lot of bankrupt businesses. For a relationship to maintain emotional intimacy and satisfying sexual expression there is an ongoing need to devote quality time, both inside and outside the bedroom.

Anger and lack of respect for your spouse can enormously drain desire. For sex to be positive in an ongoing relationship, there needs to be a sense of respect, trust, and intimacy. Anger at one's spouse, whether for sexual or nonsexual matters, festers and wears away at the marital bond. If the issue is nonsexual, the couple is strongly encouraged to deal with it directly rather than playing it out in a negative sexual scenario. If the anger revolves around a sexual issue (extramarital affairs, feeling sexually rejected, arguments over oral sex), the hurt feelings need to be directly addressed and the partners need to commit themselves to changing the problematic behavior.

Sex is often relegated to being the last thing at night after taking care of the children, watching endless TV, walking the dog, etc. Good quality sex needs an awake, aware, involved couple. Sexuality has to assume a higher priority. Being open to having sex in the morning or as a "nooner" on the weekend can go a long way toward restoring sexual desire.

Paul and Sylvia

Paul had been a very ardent courter of Sylvia fourteen years before. At thirty-two, Paul felt ready to marry and was quite attracted to twenty-seven-year-old Sylvia. Paul had just been promoted to partner in his law firm, a goal that had taken the majority of his time and energy for the past seven years. Paul was a very energetic and goal-oriented man, and this was transformed into an intense and passionate courtship. Sylvia appreciated the attention and caring from Paul and happily entered into marriage with him. They had two daughters in five years, and much of their energy went into parenting. Paul was involved with his career, politics, golf, and parenting, and sex slipped into a Saturday-night routine. The sex was functional, but not very creative or exciting. Sylvia began experiencing increasing frustration with Paul and their marriage. She resented how little time they spent as a couple, and how little affection (except for perfunctory hello–good-bye kisses) was displayed outside the bedroom. Sylvia developed a reactive depression and reported no sexual desire for Paul. During the year previous to entering therapy, they had had intercourse only three times. Paul's approach to the sexual inactivity was passive acceptance and a marked decrease in his own desire. This was a couple in trouble and headed for more severe marital and sexual dysfunction.

To reverse this trend, Paul and Sylvia entered therapy, where regaining sexual desire was one of the integral components. The first "homework exercise" was to restart an affectionate and sensuous relationship both inside and outside the bedroom. They took turns engaging in caressing and stroking in the bedroom with clothes on and verbalizing what they were feeling. Paul was cautioned that he shouldn't try to make sex a goal-oriented work task, but rather to be an active, involved partner in the process of giving and receiving pleasure. One night, they took the children to their in-laws' and instead of going out to the movies returned to their home. They experimented with sensuous, nondemand touching in the nude while in the living room. To prevent interruptions they locked the doors and took the phone off the hook. To set a mood they put on their favorite music and used soft lighting. To enhance the sensations of touch they used a body lotion they had jointly chosen at a specialty shop. These two experiences made Paul and Sylvia aware of how much they were cheating themselves and each other by settling for a nonsexual relationship, and reignited a sense of sexual anticipation and intimacy.

Another "homework exercise" was to engage in a verbally oriented attraction experience. Sexual attraction is an ongoing process, building on the elements (physical, emotional, and interpersonal) you like about your partner. In our culture, myths about romantic love and a natural "chemical" attraction abound. The reality is that romantic love feelings seldom last more than a year or two at a maximum. They need to be replaced by a more mature love and nurtured by fulfilling emotional and sexual experiences.

Paul began by saying to Sylvia the things he found most attractive about her. This included, for instance, her sparkling green eyes, her concern for their house and children, the way she looked at him as she kissed him, her smell when she became sexually aroused. He was encouraged to spend as much time as he wanted acknowledging all the things that made her an attractive person. Sylvia was instructed to actively listen and accept the compliments, not shrug them off or say "Yes, but." Paul then had a chance to make one to three specific requests for change that would make Sylvia more attractive to him. Paul asked her to wear sexy things to bed—either a silky nightgown or his shirt with nothing else. Also, he requested that she tell him when she wanted to be sexual. Roles were then reversed, and Sylvia had a chance to acknowledge Paul's attractiveness and make requests for change.

As the exercises and experiences continued, both began having more positive anticipation, valuing their time as a couple, and having intercourse and orgasm be a part of their life and marriage.

KEYS TO INCREASING SEXUAL DESIRE

When couples get away from recriminations and see the difficulty as a shared problem, they are on the road to recovery. Instead of arguing about the past, they need to focus on developing a functional and satisfying sexual style for the present and future. Touching can occur both inside and outside the bedroom, and not all touch should or needs to lead to intercourse. Rather than worry about the frequency of intercourse, the couple can enjoy the quality of their emotional and sexual relationship. They are able to talk and laugh, sometimes plan and other times be spontaneous about sexuality. Especially important is establishing a rhythm of being sexual that is at least once a week and that reestablishes the expectation that sex will be a pleasurable and energizing part of their lives. This combination of emotional intimacy and flexibility in sensual and sexual expression is an excellent basis for building and maintaining sexual desire.

17
LEARNING EJACULATORY CONTROL

Rapid or involuntary ejaculation is the most common male sexual problem. It is estimated that approximately one out of every three men is an involuntary ejaculator. Until recently, rapid ejaculation was not considered a problem. This attitude is regrettable, for the man as well as the woman, but it is fairly easy to explain.

Men learn to be rapid ejaculators during their early sexual experiences. Among adolescent boys, for example, masturbation is a secretive, hidden activity, haunted by guilt and the fear of discovery. For this reason, most young boys try to reach orgasm as quickly as possible. In the so-called circle jerk, when a group of adolescent boys masturbate in unison, the winner in terms of being most masculine is the one who ejaculates the fastest and farthest.

This push toward rapid performance carries over to the first intercourse experience. Typically, a young man's first intercourse takes place in the back of a car in a hurried, unplanned way, or on a sofa in the girl's house with the fear that her parents may return at any moment, or with a prostitute who puts pressure on him to finish quickly so she can get on with business. Present in all these situations is not only sexual arousal but also a good deal of anxiety and an explicit demand to perform rapidly. The young man is solely concerned with proving himself sexually rather than with focusing on the sensual and pleasurable aspects of the experience. Since he has learned to associate sexual prowess with rapid ejaculation rather than with giving and receiving pleasure, he is likely to reach orgasm very quickly. First intercourse involves high expectations, high sexual excitement, anxiety, and little skill. With all these factors, it is not surprising that in their first intercourse experiences the large majority of men are rapid ejaculators. In fact, many men ejaculate before intromission. This is the major cause of unsuccessful first intercourse, and it happens to approximately one in four males. As a result of these early experiences, arousal and anxiety become closely associated. The outcome of this association is rapid ejaculation.

MISUNDERSTANDINGS ABOUT RAPID EJACULATION

Although many men learn to slow down as they become more comfortable and confident in their sexual functioning, rapid ejaculation continues to be a problem for a considerable number. This results at least partially from the fact that, until recently, rapid ejaculation was not recognized as being detrimental to the sexual fulfillment of the couple. When intercourse was seen primarily as a man's right and a woman's duty, a man had little motivation to prolong sex. Since it was believed that "nice" women did not particularly enjoy sex, a man who could get the job done quickly was someone to be admired. If his wife found intercourse unpleasant or uncomfortable, she might urge him to "get it over with." Surprisingly, this kind of thinking lingers to a pronounced degree even now, especially among men who are less aware of female sexual response and who are not accustomed to the idea that women can and should enjoy sexuality and intercourse. Men generally, and rapid ejaculators particularly, tend to be both too fast and too rough in their lovemaking. Their hurried style can be very unsatisfying to women who desire more affectionate, gentle, and sensitive pleasuring as well as prolonged intercourse. But often problems arise when a woman decides to voice her dissatisfaction.

Arguments over rapid ejaculation can create a great deal of tension in a relationship. The woman feels that the man doesn't care about her as a person or about her sexual needs, and as a result she becomes frustrated and resentful. Instead of being a shared, positive experience, sex becomes a battleground. At this point, the man might react in either of two ways, both destructive to the relationship. The first reaction is to tell his partner that she is overly demanding and that they will have sex his way or not at all. This leaves the woman bitter and sexually frustrated. Other men react by telling themselves that they are sexual failures and becoming depressed. The man avoids the source of his depression—namely, sexual activity with his partner. When he does have sex, he will try to withhold ejaculation by biting his tongue, fixing his mind on unpleasant, nonsexual thoughts, using a special anesthetizing cream on the tip of the penis, wearing two condoms, or other distracting techniques. This has the effect of reducing sexual pleasure, but does not increase ejaculatory control. When the man ejaculates he does not enjoy the experience because he is busy blaming himself for reaching orgasm too quickly. The eventual outcome of this approach is that the man no longer enjoys sexual activity and sometimes develops an erection problem as well.

EJACULATORY CONTROL AND THE WOMAN

Even those men who recognize that rapid ejaculation is a serious problem often view the situation in a distorted and self-defeating light. Their attitude assumes that rapid ejaculation is detrimental only to the woman's enjoyment and that any effort to prolong intercourse is undertaken exclusively for her sake. Many men believe that if only they had better ejaculatory control their partners would automatically become orgasmic during intercourse. In fact, there needs to be more than just prolonged intercourse in order for the woman to reach climax. Recent surveys indicate that the percentage of women who experience orgasm regularly during intercourse varies from one-third to two-thirds. Some women very much enjoy the sexual experience, including intercourse, but find it easier and more satisfying to be orgasmic during nonintercourse sex.

Contrary to popular opinion, orgasm in the female does not occur automatically as a result of prolonged intercourse. Some women enjoy sex and are orgasmic during the sexual interaction, but are never orgasmic during intercourse. Other women who can be orgasmic during intercourse find that being orgasmic through manual or oral stimulation is more satisfying, although they still enjoy the intercourse experience. This is not a sexual problem, provided that both the man and woman understand and accept it as being a question of individual style and preference. Certainly, a woman who wishes to learn to be orgasmic during intercourse will find it easier if her partner has good ejaculatory control. But a man who sets out to achieve better control solely for the woman's sake is missing the point.

EJACULATORY CONTROL FOR THE MAN

The real reason for developing ejaculatory control is that there is much more to sex than orgasm. Not that there is anything wrong with the pleasure of orgasm, but why focus on it to the exclusion of other sensual and sexual sensations? Most men are not aware of the degree of pleasure they can experience through nongenital and genital touching and how turned on they can get by slow, tender, sensuous stimulation. Also, they can enjoy the responsivity and arousal of their partner as the pleasuring progresses. Not only can prolonged intercourse be very exciting for the man, but when he does ejaculate, the orgasm can be even more pleasurable because of the long, tantalizing buildup.

In seeking to acquire better ejaculatory control, we would do best to keep our sights fixed on a happy medium rather than trying to pursue unrealistic goals. There is a tendency for attitudes about rapid ejaculation to go to extremes. In the past it was considered acceptable for a man to ejaculate soon after intromission. Today, any sexual encounter that does not last at least thirty minutes and result in multiple orgasms for the woman is considered a failure by the "sexually sophisticated." This performance-oriented approach is bound to cause sexual problems. The proper association is between "sex" and "pleasure," not "sex" and "performance." When sex is viewed as a performance, you are halfway to developing sexual dysfunction.

What exactly constitutes rapid ejaculation? How soon is too soon? Obviously, there are degrees of rapid ejaculation and degrees of ejaculatory control. A man is clearly a rapid ejaculator if he ejaculates before intromission, at intromission, or within seconds of intromission. But beyond this, it is very difficult to assign a definite time limit to mark the point at which ejaculation is too rapid. Research indicates that the average length of intercourse is two to four minutes. Can we say that ejaculation after only one minute is too rapid? Thirty seconds? Fifteen seconds? Masters and Johnson have attempted to define rapid ejaculation in terms of percentages rather than amount of time. They state that if the woman is regularly orgasmic during intercourse, rapid ejaculation occurs if the man ejaculates before the woman's orgasm more than 50 percent of the time. Even this definition seems too arbitrary, however. What about the fellow who reaches orgasm before his partner only 40 percent of the time? Is it not in his best interest to seek greater control? It may be that this whole attempt at defining rapid ejaculation is on the wrong track and that the emphasis should not be on how soon is too soon but rather on helping both the man and woman gain greater enjoyment from intercourse.

LEARNING VOLUNTARY CONTROL

The central point is that if you do ejaculate more rapidly than you or your partner would like, you are experiencing a very common problem, and you will find it helpful to learn better ejaculatory control. In fact, most men would feel more comfortable with intercourse if they felt more aware and had better control over their reactions. Thus, the most reasonable and practical way to look at ejaculatory control is as a learned skill that both the man and woman can be actively involved in acquiring and that will have a good effect on the sexual enjoyment of both.

Learning ejaculatory control consists of two steps. The first is to become aware of the sensations just before the point of ejaculatory inevitability. Male sexual arousal is a voluntary response up to this point, but after it the response becomes involuntary and a man will ejaculate no matter what he or his partner does. In fact, once you have reached this point, even if your mother-in-law were to surprise you by walking into the bedroom, you would still ejaculate. Men who tune in to their sensations just before the point of ejaculatory inevitability report a feeling of intense arousal, a sense of the penis's being "full," and an urge to push forward to release the ejaculation. This occurs one to three seconds before the onset of ejaculation.

Once the man is aware of the point of ejaculatory inevitability, the second step is to develop the ability to prolong the pleasant sensations of arousal without moving to the point of ejaculatory inevitability. This strategy is the opposite of the "commonsense" approach of tuning out sexual arousal by focusing on distracting thoughts or biting on the corner of the pillow. It emphasizes instead tuning in to arousal and penile sensations and learning to monitor them.

Men who have a long-standing habit of rapid ejaculation will need to engage in a program of exercises designed to increase their ability to control the intensity of stimulation in order to prevent themselves from going beyond the point of ejaculatory inevitability. These exercises center around the "stop-start" technique, a method of controlling a man's level of sexual excitement through a simple stimulation technique. Although it is possible for a man to use this technique on himself, more effective and lasting results will usually be obtained if the woman is involved and the couple employs it as part of a program of progressive exercises. Originally, another technique, called the "squeeze," was utilized, but it has fallen into disfavor because people found it too mechanical. Using the stop-start technique is relatively straightforward, although it might take a few times before you feel comfortable with it.

EJACULATORY Control Exercises

During the first exercise, the man and woman should assume a comfortable position that allows the woman easy access to the man's genital region. She can utilize manual stimulation until he gets a firm erection. At this point she stops stimulation, causing the erection to subside. After a few seconds, the woman resumes stimulation until the penis becomes erect again, and then stops stimulation. At this stage, she is applying the stop-start technique long before the point of ejaculatory inevitability simply to get the couple used to and comfortable with the procedure.

Once this has been accomplished, the couple can move to the next step, which is for the man to employ some signal during manual stimulation to tell the woman that the point of ejaculatory inevitability is approaching. This signal can be a verbal one such as "Now" or "Okay," or he may simply motion with his hand. In any case, he should signal as soon as he feels the signs of approaching ejaculation, and the woman immediately ceases stimulation. The man should at no time try to fight down his urge to ejaculate by himself or attempt to detach himself from his feelings of arousal. He can accept and enjoy the stimulation given to him by his partner and rely on her to help him control his ejaculatory reflex by stopping stimulation. The cessation of stimulation will decrease his urge to ejaculate. They can continue to use these arousal and stop procedures for about fifteen minutes, even if they have to stop and start ten times. When the man does ejaculate, even if it is earlier than he wants, he need not be upset, but simply relax and allow himself to enjoy the ejaculation.

This is true for all the exercises. If you make what you consider a "mistake" and ejaculate, don't feel as if you have failed or done something wrong, just enjoy the ejaculation. The experience can be instructive as well as pleasurable, since it helps you learn to determine the point of ejaculatory inevitability. There is nothing magic in the stop-start technique; it is a learning process that helps you to focus more attentively on your pattern of arousal and to break the connection between arousal and anxiety. You want to maintain the high arousal, but combined with a new sense of awareness and comfort.

After the couple has finished practicing the stop-start technique and he has ejaculated, they can end their session with the man assuming the role of giver and the woman that of recipient. She can guide him in using whatever form of stimulation she finds particularly arousing and satisfying.

When the couple has done this exercise long enough to feel thoroughly comfortable with it, they can move on to the next stage. This time, the woman assumes the female-on-top position, with her buttocks resting on the man's thighs. She stimulates him, but instead of just using her hands, she may rub his penis against her vulva, although she should not insert the penis into the vagina. As soon as the man feels the point of ejaculatory inevitability approaching, he immediately signals her, and she stops stimulation. The couple can experiment with various kinds of stimulation until they feel comfortable and confident with this stage of the exercise. For example, the woman might try rubbing the penis against her breasts and nipples, or they might use oral-genital stimulation.

The final stage involves integrating ejaculatory control during intercourse. The female-on-top position is used. The woman can initiate and guide intromission in a slow, comfortable manner. After intromission, the man lies quietly and focuses on the sensations of vaginal containment. This is called the "quiet vagina" technique. He simply enjoys the sensations of intravaginal containment with no performance pressure. After a while, the woman begins slow, rhythmic, nondemanding thrusting. As soon as the man feels the point of ejaculatory inevitability approaching, he signals, and the woman stops movement. In this way, it should be possible to prolong intercourse for ten to fifteen minutes. As greater comfort and control are achieved, the couple can experiment with more prolonged thrusting and with the man controlling the coital thrusting.

Learning ejaculatory control is a gradual process. Ejaculatory control is most difficult with short, rapid thrusting in the male-on-top position. I suggest couples first establish ejaculatory control with other intercourse positions and the use of longer, slower stroking before moving to man-on-top intercourse. It is a good idea to continue using the stop-start technique occasionally for at least six months, even after the initial problem has been overcome. In this way, you can gain even greater comfort and skill at prolonging and enjoying intercourse.

Alex

Rapid ejaculation is actually one of the easier sexual dysfunctions to deal with. The stop-start technique is, for most men, a simple and effective method for gaining ejaculatory control. However, men who have been rapid ejaculators for a long period of time find it hard to believe that they can ever overcome their problem. One of my clients, Alex, a thirty-nine-year-old man in his second marriage, was a rapid ejaculator who had a poor attitude when he came to see me. His first wife had not complained about his rapid ejaculation, so he ignored the problem during that marriage. Initially, his second wife said nothing, but her resentment built. It came out six months after they were married in a blistering attack in which she claimed that Alex was selfish, inconsiderate, and cared nothing for her as a person or about her sexual needs. Alex was stunned. His wife's accusations depressed him. He felt wounded and angry at having these demands thrown at him. Most of all, he felt a sense of hopelessness; he realized that he had been a rapid ejaculator all his life and felt that it was too late for him to change.

When his wife suggested that he try professional therapy, he refused, saying that he was not the kind of person who went to therapy. Soon afterward, however, they heard about sex therapy for couples, and Alex felt this would be less objectionable. The recommendation of an acquaintance brought them to me, and we began working on the problem. As treatment progressed, it became clear that part of Alex's anxiety was caused by his reluctance to tell a male therapist that he needed help. Once he accepted the idea that learning ejaculatory control was like learning any other skill, and that he and his wife would approach the problem as a couple, he felt better about the therapy process and he became more open and cooperative.

Alex realized that learning ejaculatory control was enjoyable as well as beneficial. He and his wife found that the exercises were effective, and Alex was amazed to discover that a problem that had been with him for so long could be overcome. However, he wanted things to progress more rapidly than they did. This is a common male complaint. Men want immediate results instead of enjoying the gradual process of engaging in the pleasuring, communicating with a partner, and gaining comfort and confidence.

Alex offers a good example of the value of using a therapist in such a situation rather than trying to do it on your own. A good professional can provide guidance, help to keep the couple on track, monitor problems that arise with the exercises, and support the couple in dealing with anxiety or discouragement. The therapist will encourage the couple to maintain a regular rhythm of intercourse. If you only have intercourse once a week or less it is difficult to learn to maintain ejaculatory control.

MALES WITHOUT PARTNERS

So far, we have been speaking exclusively about men who have wives or partners who are willing to work with them to overcome the dysfunction. What about the single man who is a rapid ejaculator and does not have a regular partner?

Although it may take longer for him to learn ejaculatory control, it is possible for the male to do something about the problem on his own. He can use the stop-start technique himself while masturbating, stimulating himself to the point of ejaculatory inevitability and then stopping. He does this for fifteen minutes before finally ejaculating. This can be effective in breaking the connection between arousal and anxiety. However, the single man should not be surprised or disappointed if the control he has achieved in masturbation does not have an immediate effect on his sexual interactions with partners. There are many more emotional and interpersonal factors in a couple situation, and these tend to complicate the task of putting his newly learned skill into practice. However, if he is open with the woman and it is an ongoing, cooperative relationship, his ejaculatory control will typically improve with time.

It is worth noting that the majority of men ejaculate rapidly in their first intercourse attempt. But a man (or the woman involved) who has this experience should not take it as a sign that he is selfish, or that he doesn't care for his partner, or that he is a sexual failure. Rather, he needs to understand that his control will get better if he and his partner continue to communicate and focus on improving the pleasure experienced during intercourse. He might try spending more time on tender and slow pleasuring, concentrating less on intercourse and orgasm. If he continues to ejaculate rapidly, he should not disparage himself, but continue to enjoy the orgasmic experience. He needs to be aware that sex does not necessarily end with his ejaculation. He can continue to stimulate his partner and bring her to orgasm manually or orally. An orgasm brought about in this way can be just as enjoyable for the woman as one that occurs during intercourse, and there is no reason for the man to feel that he is any less masculine because he has given pleasure with his tongue or fingers rather than his penis.

CLOSING THOUGHTS

Learning ejaculatory control is much like learning any other new skill. You first have to decide that you want to learn it and keep your motivation high enough to go through the steps to achieve it. Realize it takes time and practice and you need not become angry or discouraged if you do not notice an immediate improvement. Since it is something you learn as a couple, you need to work together, support each other, communicate clearly, and avoid falling into the trap of blaming each other for an unsuccessful experience. In learning ejaculatory control you are not only learning a specific skill, you are also learning to communicate better about sexuality and to widen the scope of your sexual activity. You can use your increased ability to control ejaculation to make sexual activity more pleasurable for you as an individual and as a couple.

18
AROUSAL AND ERECTION

Chronic difficulty with achieving or maintaining an erection is one of the most psychologically destructive and painful experiences a man can undergo. The term traditionally used indicates how devastating the condition is felt to be: *impotence*—without potency, without strength. A man might be able to operate a jackhammer or supervise an office staff, but if his penis does not become stiff when he wants it to, he is considered a weakling, a sexual cripple. Worse yet, he considers himself in this way. He denigrates himself, ignoring his own attributes and accomplishments, convinced that anyone suffering from erectile dysfunction cannot be a real man or a successful person. The term *erectile dysfunction* is preferable to *impotence* because it's more descriptive of the problem without the emotion-laden concept of impotency. It's the penis, not the individual, that is malfunctioning. It has been rightly noted that a male puts too much of his self-esteem in his penis.

There is no good reason why erectile dysfunction should strike such terror in the male heart. Not that there is any easy or miracle cure for recurring erectile problems—there isn't, although the great majority of men can and do learn to regain their erectile functioning. The point is that erectile dysfunction is not the sexual death sentence it is portrayed to be. In fact, erectile dysfunction is an extremely common condition. By age forty, 90 percent of men will have experienced at least one occasion when they could not get or maintain an erection sufficient for intercourse. For the majority of men, it is a temporary state, a rare and atypical occurrence. For one-third of males, the

207

erection problems last longer, a few weeks or months, but eventually normal erectile functioning returns. Perhaps 10 to 15 percent of men suffer with intermittent or chronic erectile dysfunction. In the majority of these cases the cause of the problem is primarily psychological rather than medical. The reason the condition becomes severe is that, like any psychological problem, it can become self-perpetuating. Erectile dysfunction becomes more chronic and severe with time because it feeds on the performance anxiety it produces.

The performance anxiety responsible for perpetuating erectile problems, however irrational, is nevertheless extremely real. It does little good to tell the man suffering from erection problems that it's all in his head. What he needs is help in regaining feelings of confidence sexually. The first thing he needs to do is be aware of the information available on the subject. So, let us begin by considering some of the realities of male sexual arousal and erection.

FACTS ABOUT ERECTION PROBLEMS

When we speak of erection problems, we mean either the inability to obtain an erection or the inability to keep an erection sufficient for engaging in intercourse. The problem is categorized as either primary or secondary—the latter by far the more common. A male with secondary erectile dysfunction is one who has had at least one successful intercourse experience. Most men have had successful intercourse a great many times, but then begin having intermittent episodes in which they either cannot obtain an erection or, more commonly, they achieve an erection and then lose it, typically just prior to intromission. The male with primary erectile dysfunction has never had a successful intercourse experience—a rarer condition, but more frequently than is commonly believed. He usually is able to masturbate to orgasm, however, and is often able to achieve erections and orgasm through manual or oral stimulation. The man feels humiliated and embarrassed about his sexual problem and sees it as evidence of his inadequacy as a person. He needs to realize that there is more to him and to his sexuality than just the state of his penis.

Arousal and erection are not the automatic results of an erotic stimulus. Rather, a man becomes aroused when he is feeling comfortable with himself and his partner and is enjoying the pleasure of their interaction. Feelings of sensuousness set the stage for sexual excitement and erection, and then for a desire for intercourse and orgasm. An erection is not a voluntary occurrence. A man cannot force himself to obtain one. In fact, the more he wills himself to get an erection and focuses his attention on the state of the penis, the less likely is his success. Erection is the end result of a chain of psychological and physiological events. If there are links in the chain that are missing, erection will not occur. Erection is a natural physiological response that can be blocked by a number of factors, including performance anxiety, anger, depression, fatigue, alcohol, medication side effects, and so on.

When an erection fails to happen, the problem usually lies at the very beginning of the sexual response cycle. The man might be tired, depressed, frustrated, preoccupied, or just not very interested in sex at the moment. By trying to have intercourse anyway—to oblige his partner or because he thinks it is expected of him—he is going against his own needs and desires. So it follows that he will not feel very comfortable in the situation. Nor will he be very receptive to erotic stimuli. Inability to have or maintain an erection under these circumstances is altogether natural and understandable.

A different situation occurs when a man has had too much to drink—one of the most common causes of erectile problems. Although an inebriated man may feel amorous and uninhibited, his physiological sexual functioning is impaired. Men who experience erectile dysfunction after drinking heavily become anxious about their ability to perform. This anxiety may lead to their being unable to get or maintain erections on later occasions, even when they are sober.

Benjamin

This is exactly what happened to a client of mine named Benjamin, a successful forty-six-year-old salesman for a boatbuilding concern. Benjamin had always been a fairly heavy drinker, but during one period in his life when there was an increase of pressure on the job, combined with trouble with his teenage son, he began to consume more liquor than he was able to handle. On one occasion, Benjamin became quite drunk at a party, and when he and his wife arrived home, he tried to make love to her. He was unable to get an erection, and even though his wife understood it was because of the alcohol he had consumed, the episode worried and depressed him. When he attempted to have intercourse with her the next day while cold sober, he initially achieved an erection but was unable to maintain it. This pattern continued. A few times he was able to maintain an erection and function successfully, but most of the time he could not. Eventually, he stopped attempting sex with his wife altogether.

Benjamin's initial erectile problem resulted from a combination of alcohol and personal and business pressures, but at the time he was unable to see it from this perspective. The drinking became so out of control that he was forced to admit that he was becoming an alcoholic. With the aid of Alcoholics Anonymous, he managed to give up drinking completely, but his erection problem remained. It is not at all unusual, even when the initial problem is resolved, that the erectile problem continues because of performance anxiety.

It was at this point that Benjamin and his wife came to see me. At first he was quite negative and appeared to have all but given up hope of ever regaining erectile functioning. Eventually, however, he began to see that erection problems feed on anxiety. He and his wife began doing nongenital and genital pleasuring exercises for the purpose of increasing comfort and arousal. There was a temporary prohibition on intercourse so as to reduce performance anxiety. Benjamin responded well to this treatment, and in a matter of weeks he was getting more frequent erections.

AUTOMATIC ERECTIONS

The majority of men respond to an erectile problem just as Benjamin did. They ignore the importance of the initial, less obvious links in the chain of sexual arousal—namely, the feelings of comfort and receptivity that start things off. They make the erroneous assumption that erection should follow automatically whenever the opportunity for sex presents itself. It is an aspect of the myth of the male machine that a "real man" can have sex anytime, anyplace, and with any woman. The most sensible response a man can have to erectile failure is to interpret it as a sign that he does not really want to have sex at the moment—just as he would interpret the lack of an appetite as a sign that he should not order a full meal. He might simply tell his partner, "I guess I'm just not in the mood right now." Or he could request that she give him a massage—something to relax him and allow him to be more receptive and responsive. He might offer to "give to her" manually or orally.

But men who experience erectile problems do not react in this way. Their most common reaction is one of panic and desperation. Rather than trying to relax and requesting his partner to use the kind of stimulation that is most sexually arousing for him, the man avoids sharing his concerns with his partner or involving her. He may try to force himself into arousal, displaying a level of passion he does not feel. If nothing seems to work, he will make futile attempts to achieve intromission with a nonerect penis. The sexual interaction ends on a note of frustration on both partners, with misunderstanding and resentment present on each side. The man feels he is a failure, so the next time he will put even more pressure on himself to "redeem his manhood" with a good sexual performance. As a result, he is even more inhibited by performance anxiety, and in this way a vicious cycle begins. He falls into a pattern of negative anticipation, failed performance, and sexual avoidance. What started as a normal occurrence is on its way to becoming a tragedy.

EFFECT ON THE RELATIONSHIP

In addition to the havoc it wreaks on the man's self-esteem, an erection problem can be extremely detrimental to a relationship. Erectile problems are usually traced to performance anxiety, misunderstanding, and lack of communication. When a man experiences problems, it is very difficult for him to explain to his partner what is happening to him. If he believes that it is a sign of masculinity to be able to perform flawlessly in every sexual encounter, then he will be filled with an overwhelming desire to cover up his failure or to find an excuse for it. Faced with this urgent need to find a scapegoat, he may try to pin the blame on his partner, letting her believe that his failure stems from the fact that he finds her unattractive or that she turns him off in some way. She may retaliate by ridiculing him for his failure to perform, and in a very short time the relationship becomes tense and hostile.

Another equally unproductive response to erection problems is for a man to make a play for his partner's sympathy. The excuse he makes to explain his erectile dysfunction is basically accurate—overwork, tiredness, pressure, distraction—only the attitude is wrong. If the woman responds as he wants her to, by showing pity and acting maternal, the situation becomes worse. For what the man has done is to substitute his partner's sympathy and concern for the sexual gratification he cannot obtain. Her pity, in effect, becomes a crutch, which makes it all the harder for him to function in the future. What he needs is not pity or sympathy or condescension, but rather a partner who is willing to see the erection problem as a mutual problem and who will work with him in regaining comfort and confidence in responding to sexual stimulation.

While we are on the subject of the woman's role in erection problems, let us consider a thesis that has gained attention in recent years—namely, that the problem is increasing as a result of the intimidating effect of the women's liberation movement. The idea is that as women become more sexually assertive and demanding, more unwilling to serve as a passive "vessel of pleasure" for male gratification, the pressure on men to perform sexually becomes so great that they feel overwhelmed, and the result is erectile failure. It is true that there has been an increase in the number of males complaining of erectile problems. Part of this is a reflection of the greater freedom to discuss sexual problems and the fact that there are now treatment programs for sexual dysfunction, which was not true a generation ago. But this does not settle the question of whether the assertive attitudes and sexual awareness espoused by the women's movement have a negative effect on male sexual satisfaction.

The best aphrodisiac is an active and involved sexual partner. The woman who is aware of her sexuality, who can make clear and direct sexual requests, and who is sexually responsive, should increase male sexual arousal. Studies have shown conclusively that the female's capacity for sexual pleasure is at least as great as the males, and there is no possible justification for denying women the opportunity to fulfill this capacity. Some men, of course, especially those who identify strongly with traditional ideas of male dominance, might be threatened by the new female demands for equality in sex.

Part of the problem is that men are not aware that on some occasions women may be more sexually responsive and orgasmic than they are. The double standard has led them to believe that it is always the man who is the aggressor in sex and the one who enjoys it more, while women are supposed to be coy and restrained. When a woman is assertive, highly responsive, and multiorgasmic, these traditionalist men feel threatened and may react by losing their erectile confidence. Other men who are more aware and flexible see the new sexual awareness among women as a healthy development, since it means that women are now motivated to become more responsive, take more initiative, and be more imaginative sex partners. These men find that a woman's greater awareness and arousal acts as a stimulant for them. In a good relationship both the man and woman can feel free to initiate and both can say no or propose an alternative. The man can learn it is his right to say no or to say he wants more time to play or needs more stimulation. The woman's initiation needs to be perceived as a request for sexual pleasure, not as a demand for sexual performance. This attitude is certainly the more logical and productive one, and if more men adopted it, there would be little cause for concern about the effects of the women's movement on male erectile functioning.

DEALING WITH AN ERECTION PROBLEM

The most urgent question of any man who has an erection problem is what to do about it. Perhaps the first step is to consult your general physician. Although erection problems are psychological in origin in the majority of cases, they can have medical causes, and it is worthwhile to have a medical evaluation. Some of the things a physician will check are external genitalia, testosterone level, vascular functioning, neurological functioning, alcohol intake, side effects of medication, and general health problems. He will also check for diabetes, a condition that can contribute to sexual problems. However, contrary to an idea that is widespread even among people in the medical profession, men who are diabetic do not necessarily develop sexual problems. I myself am diabetic, and I find that if I maintain my diet and exercise program, the condition has no effect on my sexual functioning.

If there is reason to pursue the problem further, your physician will refer you to a urologist, the doctor who has the greatest expertise in male sex difficulties, or to a sexual-medicine specialist, who will do a more thorough vascular, neurological, and hormonal assessment. Even when the cause of erection problems turns out to be primarily vascular or neurological rather than psychological, it is still possible to have orgasms and enjoy other aspects of sex without having a firm erection.

There has been a dramatic increase in the number of men who have penile prosthesis operations to enable them to have an erection and intercourse. There are basically two types of penile prostheses. The first involves the insertion of two semirigid rods in the penis so that the man always has a semierection. The second is a cylinder-based system that can be inflated for intercourse; otherwise the penis remains flaccid. The penile prothesis is an important breakthrough in the treatment of erectile dysfunction, but its use needs to be considered very carefully. It's major surgery and is irreversible, since it destroys normal erectile functioning. Many men are attracted to it as a return to automatic erections and a magical cure for all sexual problems. However, that usually is not so. The penile prosthesis does not affect desire or orgasm, and most important, it doesn't guarantee emotional satisfaction for the man or woman. If the penile prosthesis is going to be helpful in a couple's sex life, they have to discuss in detail (after a consultation with the urological surgeon) how to successfully integrate it into their lovemaking. Having an erection does not guarantee sexual desire, psychological arousal, readiness for intercourse, or the ability to reach orgasm.

There are other medical interventions, less drastic than the penile prosthesis, being developed—including penile injections and surgery to improve vascular functioning. The man and his partner need to understand the medical, psychological, and relational aspects of the erection problem and thoughtfully discuss the range of alternatives.

DEALING WITH ERECTION PROBLEMS AS A COUPLE

Chances are the physician will give you a clean bill of health, and this can motivate you to tackle the erection problem, since you are assured the obstacles you face are psychological and relational ones.

Erectile dysfunction is best thought of as a mutual problem. Although it is the man who actually has the erectile difficulty, both the man and the woman are affected by it. The couple's sexual functioning becomes less satisfactory. Since successful sexual functioning is in the best interests of both the man and the woman, finding a solution to the problem is a task for the couple. Besides, to think of it as the man's problem exclusively puts too much emphasis on the performance aspect of male sexuality. Such an attitude increases the psychological pressure experienced by the man and decreases his chances of breaking out of the vicious cycle of anxiety-perpetuated failure.

The best course of action to follow in trying to deal with an erection problem is for the man and his partner to seek professional help. A professional sex therapist can provide the objectivity and experience that are so important in helping a couple overcome this dysfunction. It is understandable, however, that many couples would be reluctant to go running to a sex therapist or psychotherapist at the first sign of a sexual problem, but would prefer to try to overcome it on their own. For such people, the following guidelines and exercises may be useful. If the erection problem is long-standing and persistent (more than six months), however, professional assistance is in order.

During sexual arousal in the male, physical and psychological stimulation results in the filling with blood (vascongestion) of the spongy erectile tissues of the penis, and with increased myotonia (muscle contraction) there is a firm erection. Either inadequate sexual stimulation or, more often, interfering thoughts and feelings can block this naturally occurring process. The key to overcoming erectile dysfunction is to increase sexual stimulation and to replace any interfering feelings with an active involvement in the experience. The way to do this is definitely not by trying harder. Potency is one area where you don't get A for effort. Trying to force an erection is, in fact, one of the most effective ways of breaking the chain of events that make up normal sexual response.

When a man tries to make his penis erect by force of will, the result is a strained and anxious focusing of attention on the penis. Because it is not humanly possible to concentrate on two things at the same time, the attention he devotes to feelings of pleasure from the sexual interaction diminishes. He becomes detached from the situation, an emotional spectator intent only upon detecting signs of arousal, yet nearly oblivious to the erotic stimuli that cause it. Sex is not a spectator sport; you have to be an active partner in giving and receiving.

ERECTILE EXERCISES

A couple can deal with an erectile problem through engaging in exercises for increasing sexual awareness. The chief cause of erection problems is performance anxiety and insecurity. The remedy is to regain your comfort and confidence with sexual expression and naturally occurring arousal and erections. You might begin by having a quiet, intimate talk over a drink or coffee, followed by a relaxing, sensuous shower. Lather each other all over, including the genitals, then dry each other off. Be sure you have time and privacy to really enjoy the experience. Go into the bedroom and get into a comfortable position for pleasuring, with the woman starting as giver and the man as recipient. She can begin stimulation by stroking his chest or thighs and gradually moving toward his genitals. The man concentrates on accepting the feelings of pleasure he is experiencing rather than on worrying about whether he is getting aroused and becoming erect. If the man is truly receptive and the woman continues to pleasure him in a sensuous, nondemand way, an erection will eventually occur. At this point, pleasuring should cease and the couple can lie comfortably together until the erection subsides.

Be aware of your feelings at this moment. How does each of you feel as the penis returns to a more flaccid state—anxious, worried, tense, angry, relieved? Gaining confidence that an erection will return after it has subsided is especially important. One of the chief psychological traps for a man with an erection problem is that as soon as he obtains an erection, he immediately feels he has to use it. This is especially true of morning erections. When the erection dissipates before intercourse, as it

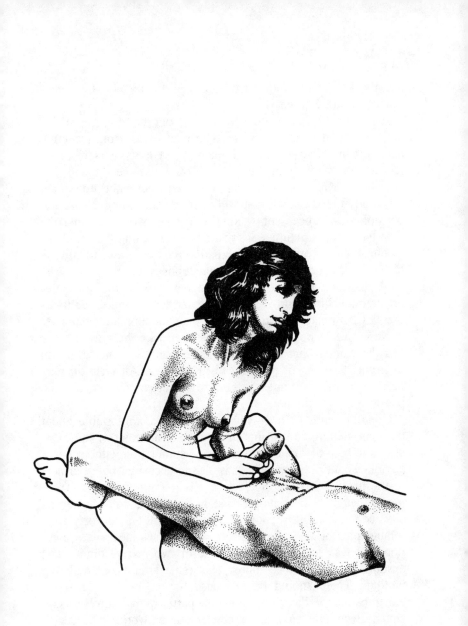

An exercise in ejaculatory control where stimulation is applied in stop-start fashion. This can counteract the tendency to premature ejaculation and prolong male and female pleasure.

usually does, he becomes frustrated and depressed—two emotions that block arousal.

After about thirty seconds the couple can return to pleasuring until a second erection occurs. The man focuses on accepting and enjoying the feelings of pleasure. Allow yourself to be receptive to stimulation. Let yourself respond to each touch. Let your body drink in each feeling. When an erection occurs, again lie quietly together until it subsides. In understanding the natural physiological process of waxing and waning of erections, the man has taken a giant step forward in overcoming the problem. Young men are used to "automatic erections" and to always having intercourse on their first erections. You can enjoy sex more and be a better lover by engaging in sensuous, pleasure-oriented touching with your intimate partner, seeing sexuality as a giving, intimate experience rather than an automatic response.

Now reverse positions, letting the man take the role of giver and the woman that of recipient. The man can concentrate on imparting feelings of pleasure to his partner. An erection may occur naturally. If it does, just enjoy the sensations and continue pleasuring your partner.

Continue until both of you have become comfortable about the man gaining and losing an erection. The point of the exercise is to help the man focus on erotic stimulation without being anxious about performance. It is also to accustom both partners to the natural process of erections. It is entirely normal for a man's penis to become alternately hard and soft during an extended pleasuring session. In fact, during a typical forty-five-minute pleasuring session before intercourse, the male's erection will wax and wane an average of two to five times. The ensuing orgasm can be more pleasurable after this tantalizing buildup. There should be no cause for anxiety or alarm for either partner if the man's erection partially or entirely disappears. Becoming anxious or concerned, or working harder to bring it back, will have a detrimental effect.

For the second exercise, the couple can use the female-on-top intercourse position. They will not actually be proceeding to intercourse during this exercise. Rather, the exercise will accustom both partners to having the penis close to and in contact with the vulva. After they are comfortable, perhaps with pillows under the woman's thighs and one under the man's head, she begins caressing and stimulating her partner. He can feel free to request specific types of stimulation and concentrate on accepting and enjoying the pleasurable sensations he is experiencing. If at any time the man becomes anxious or worried about the state of his penis, rather than retreating and having negative thoughts, he can tell his partner how he's feeling. Then, together, they can get him reinvolved in the sexual interaction. He could do this by pleasuring her or by clear and direct request for a specific kind of stimulation such as ''rub the underside of my penis with just your fingertips.''

When he gets an erection, instead of letting it subside, the woman can take the penis in her hand and rub it around her vulva area. She may use the tip of the penis to stimulate her mons, labia, and clitoris, but should not insert it into her vagina. If the man begins to lose his erection or shows signs of becoming tense, she should not stop, but rather return to fondling and caressing the penis, the testicles, and the inner thighs. She can use manual or oral stimulation, and he can feel free to stimulate her at the same time. This use of multiple stimulation, including fantasy as well as touching, is the key to building and maintaining sexual arousal. Remember, it is entirely normal for the penis to become alternately hard and soft as stimulation progresses. The exercise may end with the couple switching positions and the man pleasuring the woman, using the kind of stimulation that she enjoys most.

During the third exercise, just as an experiment, the couple can see how ineffective it is for the man to try to keep an erection, compared with the techniques they have been using in the previous exercises. The couple can use any pleasuring position they want, with the woman stimulating the man until he gets an erection. Then she should let him try to maintain the erection on his own by focusing his attention on it. Almost inevitably, the erection will be lost. Both partners should take note of their feelings at this time. The man can notice how he has become a spectator of his own reactions and how little pleasure or stimulation there is in that role. He is concerned with himself rather than being actively involved with the woman and the pleasurable, arousing interaction. The woman can notice how anxious and left out she feels as her partner tries to maintain his erection without her participation.

After they have seen the pitfalls in trying to maintain an erection through willpower, the couple can move on to the positive part of the exercise. Taking the female-on-top position again, the woman uses a variety of pleasuring techniques. She can rub the tip of the penis around her vulva area as in the last exercise, but eventually she can insert the penis into her vagina. Intromission should be initiated and guided entirely by the woman. The man lies back and enjoys himself. If she notices any tension from him or loss of erection she can resume manual or oral stimulation. Intercourse is not separate from the sensual and sexual process—it's not the pass-fail test of sex. Intercourse is best conceptualized as a special pleasuring technique; a natural extension of the pleasuring, not separate from it.

Both the man and the woman should be aware that a strong, firm erection is not necessary for intromission. With the woman's guidance and active participation, a semierect penis is relatively easy to insert into the vagina. It is a good idea for the woman to initiate the moment of intercourse and to guide the penis into her vagina. This takes the pressure off the man, and since she is the expert on her own sexuality, it is reasonable for her to guide his penis into her vagina.

When intromission has been achieved, the couple can initially confine themselves to slow, rhythmic, nondemand thrusting. There may be a tendency to thrust vigorously to try to prevent loss of the erection, but avoid this. Allow the intercourse to be involving and rhythmic. The couple can proceed to orgasm if they wish, but the major focus is on experiencing and accepting the pleasurable sensations of intercourse. Later, the couple can try other intercourse positions. They can experiment with "quickies" and can take turns guiding intromission and setting the pace of the coital thrusting.

REGAINING ERECTILE CONFIDENCE

Erection is a natural result of receptive, sexual stimulation—provided nothing blocks the chain of events that lead to arousal. The basis of erectile response is pleasure and receptivity, not performance and self-consciousness. One of the most effective ways to block arousal is for the man to give way to anxiety and to try to will an erection, thus becoming a spectator in the sexual interaction. It is crucial that he remain actively involved in the sexual experience.

Second, there must be sensual and sexual stimulation. Men who are performance oriented rather than pleasure oriented have a great deal of trouble getting themselves to request specific kinds of stimulation. Faced with erectile difficulties, they are likely to remain silent, struggling with the problems themselves, rather than saying something like "Honey, I really want to make love with you, but I'm a little out of it right now. Could you gently caress my penis the way you did last Thursday?" A person can't have intercourse alone, and neither can he deal with the erectile problem alone. The key is the one-two punch of nondemand pleasuring followed by multiple stimulation. Sexuality is an intimate form of communication. Erection problems occur when there is a breakdown in communication because one partner is tired, worried, preoccupied, or distressed. The way to deal with erection problems, or any sexual dysfunction, is to reestablish communication, to focus on pleasuring, and to see erection and intercourse as natural extensions of the pleasuring process.

19
OVERCOMING EJACULATORY INHIBITION

Ejaculatory inhibition—the inability to ejaculate with a partner—has the reputation of being a rather rare and exotic sexual disorder. Hence, the problem is usually given short shift. While it is true that ejaculatory inhibitions is much less common than either erectile dysfunction or rapid ejaculation, it is a problem that confronts perhaps 5 to 10% of males sometime in their lives. There are several different forms of ejaculatory inhibition—from the total inability to ejaculate to the specific inability to ejaculate in the vagina, with the most common type being the intermittent difficulty in ejaculating experienced by middle-years men.

A man who experiences ejaculatory inhibition typically is able to be aroused, develops and maintains an erection, but does not reach orgasm. When this occurs at rare intervals, the effect is frustrating, baffling, and anxiety producing; but for most men the ability to ejaculate soon returns. A man with severe ejaculatory inhibition is able to reach orgasm during masturbation but not with a partner, even though he may feel highly aroused. Some men only have this problem during intercourse, but others are unable to ejaculate even when their partner employs manual or oral stimulation. Oddly enough, although this condition can have acute psychological and, in many cases, physical effects, it is not taken very seriously by either experts or by the general public. Let us examine why this might be so.

CONFUSION ABOUT EJACULATORY INHIBITION

First, however, there is the matter of terminology. Since ejaculatory inhibition has not been studied as extensively as other sexual dysfunctions, there is less consensus about its basic characteristics. This uncertainty is reflected in the variety of terms that have been used by different writers to describe the condition. It has been called by several different titles in various clinical texts, including "ejaculatory incompetence," "retarded ejaculation," and "ejaculatory inability." "Ejaculatory inhibition" is preferable, however, because it is the least value laden and most accurately describes the problem. The inability to ejaculate usually stems from some type of inhibition—the inability to let go, to fully enjoy sexual arousal, and to allow it to naturally culminate in orgasm. Ejaculatory inhibition is not to be confused with retrograde ejaculation, a physiological condition in which orgasm does occur, but the semen goes into the bladder rather than being ejaculated from the penis. It is also not to be confused with the naturally occurring phenomenon in men over sixty of a lessened need to ejaculate at each sexual opportunity. Thus, ejaculatory inhibition is the problem of the male who is aroused and desires to ejaculate, but is unable to do so.

The reason ejaculatory inhibition has received so little attention can be traced to two widespread and inaccurate assumptions. The first is that ejaculatory inhibition is a problem only when it occurs in its most severe form. The second is that the man with ejaculatory inhibition, because of his great "lasting power," is able to satisfy his partner to an extraordinary degree, and, therefore, while he may miss the pleasure of orgasm, at least he has the consolation of knowing that he is a superlative lover. We might call this the "blessing in disguise" assumption.

The trouble with the first assumption is that it tends to discount the instances in which ejaculatory inhibition is associated with some other type of sexual problem. For example, in most cases of ejaculatory inhibition, the man may have an erection and begin intercourse, but even with continued coital thrusting and a high level of sexual arousal he is unable to reach climax. As he becomes more and more frustrated and more and more focused on the ejaculatory performance, his level of arousal declines, and eventually he loses his erection. "Ah ha," he says, "I have an erection problem!" But because of the lack of attention paid to the problem of ejaculatory inhibition, he is likely to ignore it as the underlying cause of his erectile problem. In other cases, a man suffering from intermittent ejaculatory inhibition might push himself so hard to reach orgasm and focus so narrowly on maintaining his level of arousal that, while he does manage to ejaculate, neither intercourse nor ejaculation holds much pleasure for him (or his partner). The probable result? Waning interest in sex. But again, because of his unfamiliarity with the fundamental problem of ejaculatory inhibition, he may not realize that it is central to his lack of sexual desire and satisfaction. The common element in each of these variations is that the natural rhythm of moving from high sexual arousal to orgasm is inhibited, and as a result, the man looks forward to and enjoys climax less. Rather than orgasm's being the natural culmination of an enjoyable and arousing sexual experience, it becomes an anxiety-provoking goal that he often fails to achieve.

The second assumption—the "blessing in disguise"—represents the male glorification of performance over pleasure in its most extreme form. What it entirely overlooks is that mutual pleasure is the key to true sexual satisfaction for a couple. Since ejaculatory inhibition greatly decreases pleasure for the man, it follows that there can be little real satisfaction for either partner. The first few times it happens the woman might be pleasantly surprised by her partner's intercourse; she may find that she is very orgasmic with such prolonged penile stimulation. However, unless she is totally oblivious to her partner, she will soon become aware of his frustration. If intercourse continues for over half an hour and the man still has not ejaculated, he will experience physical discomfort as a result of the continued high level of vasocongestion. This condition, commonly known as "blue balls," is not actually harmful, but it is acutely uncomfortable. The woman, too, usually finds prolonged intercourse physically painful.

CAUSES OF EJACULATORY INHIBITION

The causes of ejaculatory inhibition are many and varied, depending on the life experience of the man. In general, they appear to be psychological rather than physical, and usually

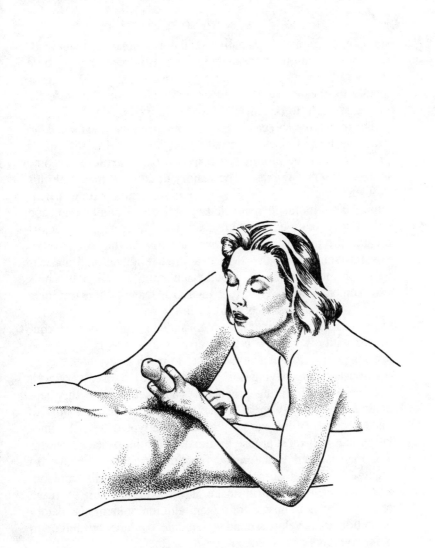

Arousal and erection are not just the automatic responses to erotic stimuli. They are also expressions of feeling comfortable with oneself and one's partner.

stem either from some negative sexual experience or from inadequate or inappropriate sexual learning. However, it is possible for there to be a physiological cause, particularly if the man is unable to ejaculate under any circumstances. In such cases, a urologist ought to be consulted to determined medical factors.

The most typical cause is that the man has developed an irrational fear of ejaculating within the vagina or in a woman's presence, and the ejaculatory response has, therefore, become more and more inhibited. The major attitude that men with this problem have is the belief that there is something wrong, frightening, or immoral in really letting go, being uninhibited, and enjoying sexual pleasure with a woman. Other negative factors include the fear of being discovered while having sex, fear or misunderstanding of the vagina, a strict religious (and antisexual) upbringing, anxiety about ejaculation, aversion to one's own semen, guilt over sexual pleasure, fear of intimacy, or a severely traumatic sexual incident in the past.

In married men, intermittent ejaculatory inhibition is connected with a tendency to think of martial sex as being routine and unexciting. If a man expects not to reach a very high degree of arousal while having sex with his wife, it may very well become a self-fulfilling prophecy. The likelihood of this happening is especially great if the man has not learned how to make requests of his partner regarding the type of sexual stimulation that will most arouse him and help him to reach orgasm. The man is used to automatic functioning and not needing to request additional stimulation from his partner. His boredom and lack of involvement make it difficult for him to reach orgasm. It is not unusual for a man with intermittent ejaculatory inhibition to develop secondary erectile dysfunction and/or to being avoiding sexual encounters altogether.

Jack

Men suffering from ejaculatory inhibition are excellent examples of the fact that in order to have a truly rewarding sex life a person must learn to please himself as well as his partner. Take Jack, a client of mine, a thirty-eight-year-old technical writer whose three children from two previous marriages lived with him. Jack seemed generally well adjusted, led an active, stimulating life, enjoyed being a single father, and reported that he had good relationships with women. But while he always experienced orgasm when he masturbated, Jack found that he was ejaculating less and less often in his sexual encounters with females. He consoled himself with the "blessing in disguise" theory that even if he was missing out on orgasm, at least he was a good lover, since his partners were nearly always orgasmic. During therapy, it emerged that Jack felt it to be unmanly for him to request stimulation from his partner. Instead, he focused most of his attention and energy on making sure that he was performing well, so his partner could have no cause to complain about his ability to satisfy her. As a result, he never got very excited during sex. As soon as he had an erection he initiated intercourse. Erection signifies a physiological readiness for intercourse, but often the man is not as emotionally and sexually aroused as he could be. Jack felt it "selfish" and "immature" to request additional penile stimulation. He never really let himself go or allowed himself to become an involved participant. Jack had made himself into a kind of "sexual servant" who was not entitled to enjoy the experience himself. We worked on helping Jack learn to request specific kinds of stimulation from his partner. He found oral stimulation particularly arousing when he was moving rather than remaining passive. He found that it was especially stimulating when his partner moved her pelvis in a circular manner during intercourse and when she stroked and fondled his testicles. As he became more confident about making specific requests, and as he gave himself permission to let go and enjoy the experience, Jack began to experience orgasm more and more regularly.

STRATEGIES IN OVERCOMING EJACULATORY INHIBITION

The major strategy in working with a man suffering from ejaculatory inhibition is to give him support and permission to enjoy and to view ejaculation as a natural and positive culmination of sexual pleasure and arousal. Like other sexual problems, the ideal is for the couple to see it as "their" problem rather than "his" problem and to work together in a supportive way to learn to be freer and more comfortable with sexual pleasure and making sexual requests. Treating ejaculatory inhibition is a gradual process in which the man allows himself to be more direct in requesting stimulation and in experiencing and savoring good sexual feelings. As he gains confidence and allows himself to become more "selfish," he will be able to enjoy the feeling of growing arousal and allow it to culminate in orgasm. The two key elements in overcoming ejaculatory inhibition are requesting multiple stimulation and being aware of orgasmic triggers. Examples of multiple stimulation include using fantasy during partner sex, testicle stimulation during intercourse, stimulating your partner's breast and anal area while she's stimulating you, so that her arousal adds to yours, kissing and stroking during intercourse, and so on. Orgasm triggers are very individualistic and are often identified during masturbation, where the man has more control. Examples of orgasm triggers include tensing leg and buttock muscles, increasing rhythm of thrusting, focusing on a highly arousing fantasy, and verbalizing how good it feels.

While gaining the ability to ejaculate intravaginally is the ultimate aim of a man wishing to overcome ejaculatory inhibition, it is generally more effective to lead up to this goal gradually. An important first step is for the man to be comfortable reaching an orgasm and ejaculating with his partner present. Letting go and lowering inhibitions by allowing yourself to ejaculate in front of your partner as a response to her manual or oral stimulation is not only normal but also a very positive step in learning to overcome ejaculatory inhibition. After you are comfortable with this, subsequent steps include relearning that sexual arousal usually culminates in orgasm and sexual satisfaction for the male, and continuing to regularly ejaculate when your partner uses manual or oral stimulation. The next step would be to begin ejaculating closer and closer to the woman's vagina in order to reduce anxiety and inhibitions related to the vagina. As the man feels less inhibited and more comfortable with regular ejaculations near the vagina, the couple can use intercourse as a major stimulation to ejaculation. The man should be aware of and request the type of intercourse stimulation that is most arousing. For example, the woman's slow and extended coital thrusting might be arousing for one man, while another might prefer the woman to be passive while he moves in short, rapid strokes. The couple can use manual or oral stimulation until the man is very aroused, and then begin intercourse. Men who enjoy multiple stimulation during nonintercourse sex typically find that multiple stimulation during intercourse very much enhances the intercourse experience. There is a cultural myth that a man should only need intercourse stimulation. Perhaps that's true of twenty-year-old men, but it's not true for the majority of fifty-year-old men. Most men in their thirties and forties would find sex more arousing if they engaged in multiple stimulation. During intercourse the man can enjoy and attend to all his feelings and sensations as well as the responses and feelings of his partner. The couple work together to reduce anxiety and inhibitions so that the man learns to feel comfortable when he ejaculates intravaginally. Remember, this is a joint effort, with the male and female working together toward a mutually satisfying sexual interaction in which arousal naturally culminates in orgasm.

Rather than trying to follow such a program on their own, many couples will want to consult a professional sex therapist or psychotherapist to help them learn or relearn these freer, less inhibited attitudes, feelings, and behaviors. If the man does not have a regular sex partner to help him, he might be particularly interested in consulting a therapist not only to help understand ejaculatory inhibition, but also to develop an individual program that will aid in reducing his anxiety and make him feel less inhibited sexually.

HELPFUL ATTITUDES

As is true with other sexual problems, the man suffering from ejaculatory inhibition needs to understand his sexual behavior, accept it without feeling less masculine, and with the help and cooperation of his partner and/or a professional therapist work toward greater comfort and more enjoyable sexual functioning. It is important to note that, just as with erectile difficulty or rapid ejaculation, a man might experience ejaculatory inhibition as a once-in-a-while thing without its being a sign that there is anything basically wrong with his sexual functioning. Any situation or feeling that interferes with free-flowing sexuality can occasionally prevent the male from ejaculating. For instance, if he is tired, if he has drunk too much, if he is depressed, if he is angry with his partner, if the sexual activity is unexpectedly interrupted by a phone call or children's demands, he might feel no need or desire to ejaculate.

Nor should the problem of ejaculatory inhibition be confused with the normally occurring decrease of ejaculatory frequency in older men. As a man reaches sixty and beyond, it is not at all unusual for him to be having and enjoying intercourse, but to feel no need to carry each encounter through to ejaculation. For instance, an older man who has intercourse five times a month may feel the need to ejaculate on only three or four of those occasions. Many older men do not understand that this is a healthy and normal part of aging, and instead feel that they're "over the hill" sexually or that they have developed a sexual dysfunction.

The important point that men need to keep in mind about ejaculatory inhibition is that it is neither a catastrophe making the end of one's sexual life nor something to be shrugged off or disregarded. It is a sexual dysfunction that, like other dysfunctions, is worth taking the time and effort to change. In most cases, ejaculatory inhibition responds readily to treatment. If you are one of the men troubled by this problem, you owe it to yourself and your sexual relationship to reestablish comfort and confidence with reaching orgasm and ejaculating.

20
A COST-BENEFIT APPROACH TO EXTRAMARITAL SEX

Compared with the sexual vistas that the single man is free to explore, marriage is a tight little world indeed. In our society, the ideal in marriage is sexual fidelity. For many men, raised on the belief that sexual conquest is the means by which a man proves his masculinity and obtains his fulfillment, the idea of being constrained to having sexual relations with one woman for the rest of his life may seem intolerable. Even when he has no real opportunity or desire for extramartial sex, a married man may still find himself obsessed by thoughts of an affair because it is forbidden and a way of demonstrating he's a "real man" and not a wimp constrained by martial bonds. Sooner or later, the chance to engage in extramarital sex will arise. And since a "real man" never turns down a sexual opportunity, it appears that an extramarital affair is something that will happen to him sooner or later, regardless of whether he actively pursues it or tries to avoid it.

MAKING CHOICES ABOUT EXTRAMARTIAL SEX
The trouble with such a fatalistic attitude, however, is that it deprives you of the power to make rational choices and take responsibility for your actions. In the case of extramarital sex, these actions may have far-reaching consequences, and so the ability to think about your values and feelings regarding marital sexuality and extramarital affairs, and to make decisions that are in your best interest, becomes extremely important. It would be worthwhile for you to look at extramarital sex in a more dis-

criminating way, to distinguish among the different levels of extramarital involvement, and to weigh the advantages and disadvantages of extramarital sex for you as a person and for your marriage.

We will try not to be influenced by the ready-made opinions and cultural stereotypes, whether they are liberal or conservative in origin. Each is liable to exert its own sort of tyranny over our thinking. One traditional attitude, for example, is that any extramarital affair, if discovered, is sufficient cause for ending the marriage. The offended spouse either leaves the house or forces the other to leave, and all communication between them ceases, except that which is carried out through their lawyers. There is another commonly accepted, traditional idea: that in any marriage the husband may be expected to have a number of brief clandestine affairs, but that the wife will remain strictly faithful and prefers not to "really know" about her husband's activities.

Some liberal-minded couples propose an entirely different attitude. An idea that gained currency some years ago was that it is not extramarital sex but sexual exclusivity that is the enemy of marriage. Monogamy restricts the individual's ability to express himself and to relate freely to others; therefore, the ideal marriage is one in which neither partner questions how the other spends his time, or with whom. According to this view, man is naturally polygamous, so "co-marital affairs," threesomes, mate-swapping, group sex—even bisexuality—can be comfortably incorporated within the marital context, provided both partners agree to give up their "selfish and old-fashioned feelings of jealousy and possessiveness." Hence, extramarital sex is seen not as a threat but as an opportunity for both partners to liberate themselves from restrictions and achieve new freedom and openness.

If we look carefully at the traditional and the "open marriage" attitudes, it becomes clear that they are equally doctrinaire, equally unsuitable as guides for real-life behavior. To see how emotional and value laden both really are, we only have to look at the contrasting terminology they employ. Those who are opposed to affairs use terms such as *adultery, cheating on your wife, being unfaithful*. Those who favor extramarital sex, on the other hand, prefer to use such terms as *personal and sexual sharing, not being hung-up by jealousy and possessiveness*, and *open marriage*. In this chapter, we will attempt to avoid both value-laden terms and judgmental attitudes. We will try to take an objective and constructive approach to the issue of extramarital sex. There is no blanket judgment—good or bad—that can apply to all extramarital affairs. Rather, each extramarital affair must be considered in the context of its meaning for the individual and his marriage situation. The individual's and the couple's religious and personal values must also be taken into account.

TYPES OF AFFAIRS

For the purpose of analysis, it is helpful to separate extramarital affairs into three basic categories: the high-opportunity–low-involvement affair, the ongoing affair, and the comparison affair. The high-opportunity–low-involvement encounter is the most common type for men. It may occur during an out-of-town business trip or as a pickup at a bar or party. Although the desire for an exciting, illicit experience or the need for sexual variety may play a considerable part in motivating a man in such a situation, the main reason most casual encounters happen is simply that it is possible for them to happen. The opportunity presents itself and there seem to be few liabilities in accepting it. Very often, these experiences are with prostitutes or at massage parlors. In the case of paid-for, impersonal sex, the man often wants to engage in a sexual activity with the prostitute that his wife is unwilling to engage in or that he feels uncomfortable asking her to do. This activity is generally fellatio; in fact, it is quite common for the married clients of prostitutes to request oral-genital stimulation rather than intercourse.

There are advantages as well as disadvantages to the high-opportunity–low-involvement encounter. One advantage is that since there is little or no emotional component to this type of affair, this is the least threatening to the marital relationship. A man may feel guilt as a result of an anonymous one-night stand, but such an experience is not likely to compete on a profound emotional level with the relationship he has with his wife. In the event that the wife discovers the affair, she may feel less threatened by it than by a more serious involvement. It is possible for a casual sexual encounter to enrich the sexual relations between the man and his wife. The man might learn new techniques or acquire a new enthusiasm for sex that he can bring back into his marriage. It can provide sexual pleasure for a man who for one reason or another receives little pleasure from martial sex, as well as add an element of excitement and adventure to his life.

The disadvantages of the casual encounter include those that exist for unmarried men as well—namely, the danger of sexually transmitted disease and/or pregnancy. People who meet casually and decide to have sex often do not bother to discuss health issues or contraceptive methods. The man may assume that the woman is on the pill, or he might just not care, and the result can be an unwanted pregnancy. There is also a chance that the woman has a sexually transmitted disease, and if the encounter is truly anonymous she may not be particularly concerned about infecting her partner. If the man does contract a sexually transmitted disease, he is likely to give it to his wife, and then he faces the extremely embarrassing task of having to reveal his affair so that he can alert her to the need for medical treatment. Another disadvantage is that the man may become involved in the drinking and drug culture that often revolves around bars and prostitution.

A further disadvantage of the casual encounter is that although it may provide sexual novelty, it often detracts from the martial relationship. A man who finds his sexual excitement and variety outside the marriage does not have much motivation to try to improve the sexual interaction with his spouse. There is the danger that casual encounters or visits to massage parlors will become a habit, reinforcing a tendency that is highly detrimental to marital adjustment—namely, thinking of sex in marriage as being routine and unexciting and sex outside of marriage as being varied and adventurous. To consider one's marriage in this way not only sells short its potential for pleasure but also contributes to its deterioration.

The Ongoing Affair

The ongoing affair is the next most common form of extramarital sex for men. Such affairs are based on an understanding between a man and a woman that they will meet periodically for sex, conversation, drinks or dinner together, but little else. There is no expectation that the relationship will develop, grow more serious or more intimate. Usually intimacy or possessiveness beyond a certain point is discouraged by one or both of the partners. Examples of this kind of affair are the salesman who spends the evening with a particular woman every time his business brings him to her area of the country, the man who visits a divorced woman every week or so for a sexual liaison, the executive who is having an affair with his secretary. These affairs are often of short duration, but if they satisfy the needs of both parties and if they can be carried on without fear of detection, they may continue for years.

The ongoing affair has definite advantages. It allows for a certain degree of continuity and human contact and it provides a supplemental sexual outlet. At the same time, it does not require a major emotional commitment or the expenditure of a great deal of time or energy. While the relationship is emotionally limited, it provides a setting in which the man can talk about ideas, frustrations, and emotions he feels he cannot share with his wife. Thus, the affair furnishes not only a sexual release but a psychological one as well. If the man's marriage is irredeemable, yet he does not wish to get a divorce, this type of affair helps him maintain appearances. The ongoing affair assuages his loneliness as well as meets his sexual needs. There is also the advantage that such a relationship, though it might settle into a comfortable and familiar routine, can, at the same time, create a sense of adventure in the man's life. The experience of arranging a secret rendevous, of leading a clandestine and illicit "double life," provides a certain charm and excitement in and of itself.

The ongoing affair has the same disadvantages as the casual encounter—namely, the possibilities of detection, of pregnancy, and of sexually transmitted disease—but it also has some of its own. The greatest danger is that it may lead to a deeper and more personal involvement than was expected. Emotions are unpredictable, and there is no guarantee that they will remain at the level intended for them. Such unexpected emotional involvement may be mutual, or it may be one-sided. But in either case, it is sure to lead to unlooked-for complications.

Most people's lives are not geared to handling sudden emotional overloads, and the consequences of being caught between a demanding, jealous mistress and an increasingly suspicious wife may be disastrous. Since this type of affair quite often ends up consuming more time and psychological energy than originally anticipated, it can detract from other areas of a man's life. One of the first effects of the time squeeze is on his relationship with his children; he simply does not have the time to devote to the father role. He finds that he has less time for his business, hobbies, and friends. Ironically, what was originally undertaken for pleasure and recreation can end up increasing the demands and restrictions on his time and energy. Unless the man can manage to break off the affair (usually an immensely harder and more complex task than starting it), the situation may easily get out of control and could end in catastrophe.

Another disadvantage of this type of affair is the loss of intimacy with one's wife. Not only is the ongoing affair likely to have a bad effect on the man's sexual relationship with his wife, but it is also likely to affect their emotional relationship as well. The man puts less energy into his marriage and shares his thoughts and feelings less with his wife. Because of guilt and/or the fear of discovery, he is particularly guarded or uncommunicative, and, as a result, his wife may become suspicious or simply feel he no longer cares very much about her. She withdraws her intimacy and affection, causing him to turn more and more to the outside partner for personal support as well as sexual gratification.

Brian and Ellen

Brian and Ellen provided a good example of the toll that a husband's extramarital affairs can take in terms of the time and energy they consume. It was Ellen who came to see me in therapy originally. She was unhappy, dispirited, complaining that the responsibilities of caring for a home and two children left her feeling frustrated and inadequate. She reported needing some change in her life and was considering returning to school. It soon became clear that one of her main problems was that her husband was too busy to give her much help or emotional support. At my suggestion, Ellen requested that he participate in the sessions as well. After talking to the two of them together and to Brian alone, I learned the story behind their present troubles.

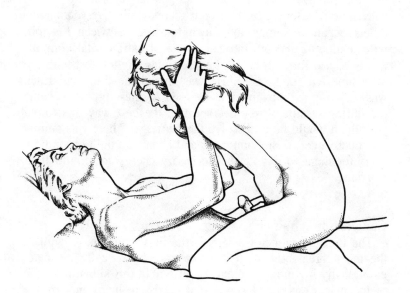

By multiple stimulation and fantasy, the man can help overcome ejaculatory inhibition.

Brian was a leasing agent who had relatively flexible hours and contact with a wide variety of people. During the first two years of marriage their sex life had been fairly good, but after Ellen became pregnant sexual relations stopped almost completely. Brian decided to seek a sexual outlet outside of his marriage and engaged in a number of casual affairs. He found extramarital sex more exciting than the "settled-down" sex he had with his wife. Brian felt he had recaptured the feelings and sense of challenge he had experienced before he was married. He enjoyed the sense of getting away with something by keeping the affairs a secret from Ellen. Brian continued in this pattern until, after the birth of their second child five years later, things began becoming too much for him. Between his job, wife, children, and the intricate circle of extramarital commitments he had formed, he felt he was living life too fast with too little time left for himself. He was spread too thin, and Ellen was suffering for it as much as he was. As these problems came out during sessions, they decided that the best way of dealing with them would be to dissolve the marriage. There was simply too much anger, disappointment, and alienation built up on both sides for them to devote the necessary energy to rebuild their marriage.

Comparison Affairs

The third category of affairs is the most complex as well as the most threatening to the status quo: the sexually intimate, emotionally involving comparison affair. In this situation, more of the man's emotional and sexual needs are being met by the affair than by his marriage. There are definite advantages as well as disadvantages to be considered in the comparison affair.

Having an intimate affair can be a powerful ego booster, particularly for someone who is feeling down about a job problem, family troubles, or just middle-age blues. If love, excitement, and passion have been missing from one's life for some time, it can be very exhilarating to feel them again. Finding that he is still capable of loving and being loved causes a man to feel that he has a new lease on life. It has been said that love is the best tonic, and this can be as true of an extramarital relationship as of any other. Having a comparison affair may have a profound regenerative effect on a man's whole life. It may galvanize him into taking things in hand in a way that he felt little motivation to do previously. For example, if a man's marriage has deteriorated beyond repair and he has been too apathetic to do anything about it, having a comparison affair can show him what he has been missing and spur him to take steps toward getting a divorce. In fact, the single most frequent cause of a man's leaving his marriage is a comparison affair.

The potential disadvantages of a comparison affair, however, can also be great. The dangers and problems associated with the other two types of affairs result from this type as well. In addition, the comparison affair has the most potential for ending disastrously. It places the greatest psychological stress on the man, since in effect he is leading two separate lives. One of the two women involved will end up feeling hurt and rejected, and there is the possibility that the man will eventually be deprived of both relationships. The emotional conflict can become intense, and it can have a wrenching effect on family, job, and sense of well-being. Most men are incapable of sustaining this kind of double life, no matter what one reads in the recent spate of books and articles advising people on how to deal with multiple love relationships. The majority of men who become involved in a comparison affair eventually find that they had to choose between the affair and the marriage. And that choice will probably be accompanied by a considerable amount of turmoil and psychological pain. The joke in mental health circles is that if people stopped having affairs it would cut business by one-third. These affairs usually throw marriages into crisis when discovered, and even if not discovered cause emotional turmoil for the man and his paramour.

A subcategory of the comparison affair is the highly romantic, emotionally intense relationship that has not been sexually consummated. The sense of the forbidden and the tantalizing fantasy of being sexual can control the person's thought process. Discussions with the woman about how they are just best friends and shouldn't get involved sexually serves to build the sexual tension. In this atmosphere, a kiss or a touch ignites powerful feelings and desires. In some ways, unconsummated affairs are a more powerful threat to a marriage than any other extramarital relationship.

TAKING RESPONSIBILITY FOR DECISIONS

There is a good deal of simplification in this discussion of the advantages and disadvantages of different types of affairs. In real life such extramarital encounter is unique and does not fit neatly into any category. No matter how carefully we enumerate the pros and cons of a given course of action, we can never balance one side against the other in any truly objective way. In the end, we choose intuitively and on the spur of the moment, often regretting this way of acting later. This is all the more reason for taking stock of our situation and our feelings beforehand so as to have some basis for future decisions. Ideally, a husband and wife, early in their marriage, would frankly and openly discuss the subject of extramarital sex in order to share and clarify their thoughts and feelings on the matter. In reality, this is seldom, if ever, done. The man usually has an implicit assumption that is often different from his spouse's. The man typically assumes that his wife won't have any affairs and that he might have a high-opportunity encounter or an ongoing affair. Few people plan to have a comparison affair.

MY PERSONAL EXPERIENCE

When Emily and I were married, part of the traditional, male chauvinist baggage I brought with me into the relationship was the assumption that I would have clandestine affairs. I hadn't thought much about Emily in relation to extramarital sex, but I assumed that she would not follow my example. After a year of marriage the subject came up in conversation, and Emily told me that she would not accept a double-standard approach to extramarital sex. One of the goals in our marital relationship was to develop and maintain a sense of personal equity. I reassured her that the only affairs I would consider would be high-opportunity–low-involvement affairs; that the affair would be nonemotional and would be kept totally apart from the marriage. She said if I could have affairs then she would reserve the right to also have affairs. Emily expressed her distaste for casual affairs, and said if she had an affair it would have some level of emotional involvement. We discussed whether I would feel comfortable about her having emotionally involving affairs with other men, and I had to admit that I wouldn't. We confronted the issue of whether we could maintain a sexual double standard in our marriage. It seemed clear that, in our case at least, a single standard would be more satisfactory, and that marital fidelity would be a better choice for me than a variety of casual affairs.

Thus, we made our feelings and expectations explicit. The advantage of this is that our agreement allows us more freedom in interacting with friends of the opposite sex than we would have if neither of us felt sure of the other's commitment. It also makes us more vulnerable to hurt if either of us does break the agreement and has an affair. If this did occur, it would cause hurt and anger and would require a good deal of talking and confrontation, but because of our strong commitment to each other, it would not necessarily be devastating for our relationship. Our agreement has so far met the needs of our marriage quite well, but it does not necessarily mean that it would be good for you or your marriage. You need to be aware of your own values, feelings, experiences, and life situation.

GUIDELINES ABOUT AFFAIRS

Besides being aware of the advantages and disadvantages of different kinds of extramarital sex, you should be aware of guidelines that can be applied in such situations. The first guideline is that the better the marriage, the less there is to be gained from having an affair. If a basically good relationship is beset with sexual or emotional problems, it makes far more sense to try to work these out together within the marriage rather than to form a new attachment and, in effect, resolve them unilaterally. If the problems seem overwhelming, then a marital therapist may be consulted. Many people reject the idea of seeking professional help because they see it as a sign of weakness, and acknowledgment that things have gotten beyond their capacity to deal with them. But if anything, the decision to consult a professional is an indication of a couple's commitment to their relationship, a sign of the value they place on it. Moreover, a therapist who has training and experience in dealing with marital and sexual problems can provide the objective viewpoint and knowledge that are needed to better understand and resolve conflicts.

Another guideline is to beware of self-deception in extramartial affairs. It is very easy to convince yourself that what you are doing is motivated by the best intentions when actually it is not. For example, where extramarital sex is concerned, honesty is not necessarily the best policy. Confessing an affair to your spouse may appear on the surface to be a virtuous act. You may feel that you are promoting an honest and open marital relationship by sharing your experiences, but what you may actually be doing is indirectly expressing hostility and/or trying to alleviate your own guilt. Living with the discomfort caused by keeping a part of your life secret from your spouse may be the price you must pay for having an affair. In most cases, it is unfair to expect a spouse to accept the knowledge of an affair and to go on with the marriage as if nothing were out of the ordinary. Having an affair and enjoying a state of innocence at the same time is simply too much to expect. One strategy sometimes employed by men in this situation—persuading their wives to have an affair of their own to "even things up"—represents a form of coercion that reflects the husband's need to assuage his guilt more than concern for the needs of his wife. It might be a roundabout and, therefore, dishonest way of expressing a desire to split up the marriage.

Finally, there are patterns that nearly always indicate that the motivation behind the affair is a dishonest and destructive one. For example, there is the man who has a series of affairs, usually with younger women, in an attempt to prove his attractiveness and sexual prowess. This man may tell himself that his wife simply does not turn him on anymore, forcing him to seek sexual gratification elsewhere, but there is a basic problem here that he is refusing to face.

Sexual dysfunction is a poor reason to seek extramarital sex. It is true that many men (and women) with a sexual dysfunction in a marriage will have an extramarital affair to see if they are functioning in the affair (that is, does he have better ejaculatory control, better erection, greater desire, or absence of ejaculatory inhibition?). However, once you have that information the issue still involves how to deal with the marital sex. The more honest and productive approach would be to try to solve the problem within the context of marriage, seeking professional sex therapy if required.

Another example of a destructive behavior is the man who repeatedly seeks extramarital encounters with married neighbors, with his wife's friends, with co-workers, and with others whose identity would make detection of the affair both extremely likely and extremely awkward. Such a man is probably using extramarital sex as a means of inflicting punishment on either himself or his wife—and possibly on both.

In cases where self-deception is not involved, extramarital sex can serve a positive role in the man's life. Like a premarital affair, an extramarital affair can be a learning experience; it may show a person what is possible in a relationship, sexually or emotionally or both. Whether the knowledge gained in extramarital sex is used to enrich the marriage or to hasten its dissolution is a matter the individual must work out for himself.

Jack

Jack, an older student in my course in human sexual behavior, wrote a personal sex history as part of a class assignment. His story illustrates the way in which extramarital sex can have a positive effect on a marriage. Jack was a twenty-nine-year-old accountant who had grown up in a fundamentalist home. He married at twenty-one, and although he had done some dating, he had never had sex with any woman besides his wife. Although he was reasonably happy with his job, house, and particularly his four-year-old son, he felt that his life was lacking in excitement. Sex with his wife was functional, but routine. Although it took him two years to admit it to himself, what he wanted was an affair. It took another six months before the opportunity arose at an out-of-town business meeting.

Although the sex that first night was not great, Jack felt tremendously free and liberated. During the next year, he sought opportunities to travel away from home and to have sexual liaisons. One woman gave him his introduction to oral sex, and when he got home he initiated his wife into this technique. After a year, Jack encouraged his wife to have an affair to "free her up sexually." They made an agreement not to talk about the details of their affairs, but would share the new sexual techniques they learned. This pattern continued for two years, and their sex life prospered.

At present Jack has no ongoing affairs because his sexual

relationship with his wife has improved so much and because there had been some emotionally draining discussions and arguments in the past, especially about Jack's reactions to his wife's affairs. However, if a really tempting opportunity presents itself for an affair when he's out of town, he won't turn it down. Their personal relationship has matured, partly due to talking about their feelings about the marriage and other relationships. Their efforts to incorporate techniques learned in extramarital relationships brought them closer together and helped to reduce some of the doubts and fears that usually accompany such affairs.

SWINGING AND OPEN MARRIAGE

Some couples claim that "swinging," the mutual exchange of sex partners, is one way of having extramarital sex without endangering the marital relationship. Couples who have tried swinging constitute about 1 to 3 percent of the married population. They assert that by having extramarital affairs under controlled conditions, they are able to inject variety and excitement into their marriages while still maintaining mutual respect and trust. There is nothing necessarily bad or deviant about swinging—it depends on the couple, their goals, their values, and the nature of the relationship. It is worth noting, however, that few couples swing for more than about six months, and that it is usually the husband who is responsible both for making the decision to swing in the first place and for calling it off.

"Open marriage," an arrangement in which each partner is free to have extramarital relationships without having to hide these activities, has been advocated in some best-selling books. However, the research studies done on open marriage strongly indicate that it is not a viable model for most couples. It's an example of something that sounds good as cocktail party chatter, but has had very negative effects on peoples' lives and marriages. There is a great potential in such relationships for both coercion and self-deception. The assumption behind open marriage is that a mature and liberated person would not feel anger and jealousy about his or her spouse's having a sexual relationship with another person. Since all of us want to believe that we are mature and liberated, we may deny having certain reactions toward our partner's extramarital affairs when, in fact, we feel them. The danger comes when these suppressed feelings suddenly burst forth, capsizing the marriage in a storm of resentment and violent emotion.

REACTIONS TO YOUR WIFE'S EXTRAMARITAL AFFAIR

Statistically, a husband is more likely to engage in extramarital sex than a wife. Kinsey found that about 50 percent of all married men had had a least one extramarital encounter, and more recent surveys indicate that the figure may be nearer 55 or 60 percent. Compared with this, between 25 and 40 percent of wives have had extramarital sex. A prime factor behind this discrepancy is that men have more opportunities for sex outside of marriage. Also, having affairs is seen as part of the male role. In addition, males are much more likely to engage in paid sexual affairs, which is very unusual for women. A usually unmentioned factor is that men are more inexperienced than women at turning down sex. A man should learn to apply logic and understanding not only to his own real or potential involvements but also to those of his wife.

Men react more strongly to their wives' extramarital affairs than women do to their husbands'. This is largely due to the sexual double standard, which assumes that men need variety and excitement in their lives while women do not. It is considered more acceptable for a man to have extramarital sex, but a woman who has an affair is regarded as being unfaithful and dishonest. This difference in attitude also reflects the kind of affairs women tend to have—the most typical female affair is a comparison affair. The casual encounter, the most common form of male extramarital sex, is rarer among women. This contrast reflects the profound and complex differences in cultural conditioning affecting the attitudes and responses of men and women. Moreover, there is support, if not outright peer pressure, for men to engage in casual affairs, while this attitude is not found in most female peer groups. Typically, the woman has an affair to fulfill important emotional and/or sexual needs she finds unsatisfied in the marriage. In other words, the wife's affair tends to be more significant in terms of its implications for the intimacy and stability of the marriage. This is the main reason men find their wives' affairs so threatening.

There is no pat strategy for dealing with the discovery of a wife's extramarital affair. However, there are some practical guidelines that might prove of value. It is part of the traditional masculine role that when a man discovers his wife is having an affair, his response must be one of vindictive rage and possibly violence. For a man to react in any other way is to compromise his sense of honor and masculinity. This reaction, socially approved as it may be, should be avoided. The fact that your wife is having an affair need not be interpreted as an insult to your masculinity. Nor is it a sure sign that the marriage is destined to end in divorce. However, it does mean that the marriage is in major trouble and that some important personal and/or sexual needs are not being met by the relationship.

Perhaps the best way to approach your wife's affair is to understand its significance in the context of the marital relationship. The affair may be, at least partially, a message drawing attention to deficits of your marriage. Her decision to have an affair may reflect her boredom and dissatisfaction with her roles as wife, mother, worker, and social organizer. It may be an expression of her feeling that you do not devote enough time and attention to her, that she is neglected and unappreciated. It also may reflect her anger at you for not seeing her as an equal partner. Obviously, there are many reasons for affairs, but two of the newer ones for women are the greater opportunity and the use of the affair as a statement of personal independence.

Men are threatened by the idea that their wives might have greater sexual satisfaction with another man than with them. This fear can be heightened if there is a sex problem in the marriage. In the majority of cases, however, it is the need for emotional and psychological satisfaction that motivates women to have extramarital affairs, not simply the desire for better sex. Thus, the question the man needs to ask himself is not "How have I failed as a sex partner?" but rather "What emotional needs have I not satisfied as a husband and lover?"

On the other hand, one should not make the mistake of interpreting a wife's affair too egocentrically, as though whatever she did could only have significance in terms of yourself. Sometimes it has to do with opportunity. Sometimes relationships deteriorate too much to be repaired. The message conveyed by the wife's affair may not be that she wants more love and attention from you, but simply that the marriage is unsatisfactory and she wants out. Then, of course, there is always the possibility that the chief reason for her affair is that she has become attracted to another man whose company she prefers to yours—not a pleasant turn of events, to be sure, but one that must be faced and dealt with should it be true. A marriage ended by an affair is particularly hard on a male, but he can be a survivor and rebuild his personal and sexual self-esteem.

CLOSING THOUGHTS

If we begin with the assumption that marriage is a potentially viable institution that can provide great rewards for the couple willing to work at enhancing the quality of their relationship, then I think that we must regard extramarital sex with a certain degree of wariness. In most cases, the effect of an extramarital affair on a marriage is negative. For the man or woman who is dissatisfied with marriage, either sexually or emotionally or both, it is more profitable to work at solving these problems within the marriage than to seek escape in a second relationship and leave the marriage hanging in midair. In and of themselves, extramarital affairs cannot be categorically judged as either bad or good, but must be understood according to how they affect the marriage and each individual involved. In certain cases, extramarital affairs may have a positive influence on a marriage, and in other cases they may serve a useful purpose in a basically flawed marital relationship. A person thinking about engaging in extramarital sex should keep in mind that there is always an element of risk, personally and maritally, in any such affairs.

21
SINGLE AGAIN

Some theorists have suggested that the laws governing marriage should be changed to conform to those that apply in business situations. Instead of making a forever commitment to marriage and putting all of your plans, finances, and sexuality into the marriage, you would sign a marriage contract that would specify limits, especially financial, and what would happen if the marriage didn't work. There would be a time limit—say, five years—after which the marriage contract could be renewed, modified, or terminated.

Such arrangements may indeed become popular with some couples in the future. But at present it is safe to say that most of us marry with the expectation, or at least the hope, that the relationship will be a source of intimacy and security for a lifetime. How many of us achieve this goal, however, is another matter. The fact is that a substantial proportion of today's marriages fail to live up to the "happily ever after" expectations with which they began. Out of every ten couples choosing wedlock today, more than four end their relationship with divorce. Although divorce is very common in our culture and is much less stigmatized now than it was a generation ago, the transition to being single again is a difficult one. It takes a lot of energy and effort to readjust psychologically, socially, and sexually to the new state. Research studies on divorce indicate that the psychological process of deciding to divorce, going through the divorce, and accepting the reality of it commonly takes at least two years.

A generation ago, unless there was a clear and overwhelming

reason to divorce (spouse or child abuse, alcoholism, lack of financial support), couples stayed together. There was strong family, community, and religious support for marriage. Many unhappy and destructive marriages were maintained because it was the easy thing to do. However, in the present, when one or both spouses feel the marital bond of respect, trust, and intimacy is weak or unfulfilling, they are likely to end the marriage. Not only is there a rise in the number of divorces, but the number of women leaving their husbands has dramatically increased. It is now estimated that 70 percent of divorces are initiated by women. Thus, the man has to deal with the situation where he is the one who is left rather than assuming the role of the one who leaves.

The divorced man must learn to accept the loss of an accustomed companion and sexual partner. No matter how poor the relations between the couple were, divorce leaves an emotional gap that can be a source of pain and grief for months. He must consider the options available to him now that he is single again and think through alternatives for the future.

A divorced man may experience considerable depression, based as much on a sense of failure as a feeling of loss. Many divorced men believe that they are failures in the eyes of family, friends, and society—that they have not lived up to the husband-father roles they undertook when they married. Rather than dwell on this sense of defeat, however, it is far more productive to view a divorce as an unfortunate but necessary step and one that can ultimately be a valuable learning experience. If there is no possibility of partners achieving satisfaction within their marriage, then divorce is a logical and psychologically healthy alternative. Many men report a feeling of relief to be out of an unsatisfying marriage. The lessons that a man can learn from such an experience, about himself as a person and the nature of marriage, can be significant and helpful in dealing with future relationships.

CHILD CUSTODY AND VISITATION

The divorced man with children has to deal with his role as father, including child-support payments and visitation rights. This is a complex subject that could take up a whole book in itself, but I would like to offer some basic guidelines. Sometimes children feel they caused the divorce—that if they had behaved differently the marriage might have been saved. You need to make it clear to the children that the problem lay not with them or with your role as parent, but rather with the relationship between yourself and your wife. It is important to stress that they should not take sides, and that although the marriage has ended, you are still their father and you care about them.

Maintaining your financial responsibilities to your children, no matter what your feelings about your ex-wife, is important for their sense of trust. Unfortunately, mothers are given custody of the children much more often than fathers. I am a strong supporter of the concept of joint custody, when feasible. No matter what the custody arrangement, it is important to be consistent and caring during visitation with your children.

Often there is a good deal of anger and bitterness between spouses, and they use the children as their battleground. This is destructive not only for the children but also for your ability to develop a new single life. Although you are likely to be angry, or at least highly ambivalent, about your ex-spouse, you need to realize that for your own sake and the children's sake, everything would go better if each of you succeeded in establishing a new life. You need to relate to each other in a respectful, cooperative manner but keep your emotional distance from each other, especially regarding new romantic relationships.

NEW RELATIONSHIPS

It can be very difficult for a man who has recently divorced to try to establish a new relationship. Particularly when the divorce involved a great deal of emotional pain, the newly single man might be unwilling to become intimate with another woman and thereby make himself vulnerable to further hurt. Still, most men find that the dangers of investing in a new relationship are outweighed by the joy and satisfaction that closeness can bring. In fact, about five out of six divorced men do remarry, typically within three years of the divorce. What happens all too frequently, however, is that the man picks a new marriage partner who is remarkably similar to the first wife and with whom the tensions and difficulties of the original marriage are repeated.

The fact that the divorce rate for second marriages is significantly higher than for first ones indicates that this pattern is widespread. Instead of falling into this trap, the divorced man should make every effort to use the unsuccessful marriage as an opportunity to learn what elements must be present to make a marriage satisfying for him. The man who wishes to remarry should take the time to seek out a truly compatible partner rather than just rush into marriage to escape the loneliness of being single. When a man uses divorce as an opportunity for learning, his second marriage is usually a more intimate and satisfying one than his first.

Jim

Jim was a divorced man of thirty-two whose first marriage had lasted five years. Although the divorce was a bitter, drawn-out one, Jim continued to function well through the turmoil, completing his master's degree in business administration. During the waiting period for the divorce, Jim had a series of affairs lasting a few months each. When the divorce became final, he decided that he had had enough of these short, primarily sexual, contacts and wanted a more intimate relationship, though not necessarily one that would evolve toward marriage.

After two unsuccessful tries, he did establish a close relationship with a divorced woman who had a young child. They lived together for two and a half years, but finally decided to separate. Jim met another woman at work and began to date her. Judy was divorced and had two children. Although their relationship became a deep and intimate one, Jim continued to live alone, having learned the dangers of establishing a living-together situation without first being clear about what was involved. Jim wanted to be sure he had entered into the affair with Judy for healthy reasons, not because he needed to escape the dating scene, avoid lonely nights, or have someone take care of him. Jim and Judy did decide to live together and later to marry, but not before thoroughly discussing their feelings and expectations. They agreed that Jim would adopt her two children and that in a year they would have a child of their own. They also discussed their sexual needs, career plans, and living arrangements, making sure in each case that the problems that had occurred in their first marriages would not be repeated in the new relationship. This planning paid off, and their marriage has proved to be a solid and satisfying one.

Social Friendships

Before establishing a new and successful sexual relationship, however, a divorced man must first be able to meet possible partners socially. Our society does not make it easy for him to do this. There is a tendency for married people to have married friends, and a newly divorced man may find that the social occasions open to him are reduced. Some married couples, unaware of the loneliness a divorced man experiences, may feel awkward about including him in their activities. Rather than expecting others to read his mind, the man who finds himself single again should take responsibility for letting his friends know his needs and feelings. Friends may feel uncomfortable discussing social possibilities and women with him, or unsure about whether and how to bring up the subject of his divorce, or they may go to the other extreme and assume he is having a great sexual time as a bachelor and tell him how much they envy him. It is up to him to be honest and straightforward and to tell them how he is doing and what he needs or doesn't need from them. He must make certain things clear, such as whether or not he objects to being invited along with his ex-wife, whether he appreciates his friends' efforts to "match him up" with unmarried women, and whether he objects to being a single person at couple get-togethers.

Sexual Friendships and Degree of Intimacy

One of the first questions you need to ask yourself is what level of intimacy in a relationship you are presently interested in. Some men are principally interested in picking someone up at a bar or party and having a series of one-night stands. Often the motivation is to reassert one's masculinity and to recover from the sense of loss. It's a way of saying you're an attractive male and can have sex with a variety of women. For most males, this is a transitory phase that soon grows stale.

The concept of a sexual friendship is appealing for many

men. This involves establishing a companionate and sexual relationship with a woman that allows for a degree of communication, emotional intimacy, and sexual sharing, but without the implicit promise that this will be a permanent union. It has the advantages of any friendship, without the pressure of making promises of marriage, permanence, or deep levels of trust and intimacy. Some sexual friendships include an agreement about exclusive dating and/or sexual exclusivity, but many do not. A sexual friendship might last two months or two years, and you might continue to be friends after you've stopped being a sexual couple. Men look back on a sexual friendship and feel good about themselves and the time spent together. Other men find the end of the sexual friendship leaves a bad taste; there are hurt feelings and a sense of being "ripped off" or "taken for a ride." This is most likely to happen when the man (or woman) has unrealistic expectations, or makes promises he or she can't keep, or tries to make the relationship more than it can be. For example, couples who move in together—or even worse, buy a house together or switch jobs or cities for the sake of the relationship—feel particularly cheated and bitter. Another common trap is for the man to become overly involved with the woman's children or for her to become a "temporary stepmother" for his children. In entering into and maintaining a sexual friendship, enjoy it for what it is and keep a realistic perspective on the degree of intimacy, trust, and permanence this kind of relationship offers. One of my favorite clinical guidelines is that a marriage should never be more than one-third of one's self-esteem; a sexual friendship is an important but transitory part of your life and should never be more than 20 percent of self-esteem. One does not make major life changes for a sexual friendship.

What about the man who is looking for a greater degree of intimacy and security and would like to find a partner to marry? First, be sure you are doing this for genuinely positive reasons— that you are aware enough to make a choice and are ready to make the emotional and sexual commitment necessary to sustain a successful marriage. After all, it's not worth the trouble to marry again unless the new relationship adds significantly to your life. You can live a fulfilling and satisfying life as a single person. Seeking to marry to alleviate loneliness, or to have a mother for your children, or to get someone to take care of you, is likely to backfire and cause more disruption in your life than remaining single. You can take care of yourself; the decision to seek out a marriage partner should be a choice to enhance emotional and sexual intimacy and security in your life.

A second guideline is to not feel desperate, but to clearly and realistically discuss issues with the new woman in your life. Some men decide that this time they are going to put more of themselves into a marriage and are so eager to marry that they make all kinds of assumptions about their new romantic partner. Rather than being swept away by romantic illusions or an unrealistic belief that this relationship is perfect because it's so much better than the prior marriage, ask yourself and your new partner the hard and important questions about a new marriage. What would your life look like five years from now? What are the special issues—about sexuality, living arrangements, finances, stepchildren, whether to have additional children, dealing with family and friends, and so forth that need to be talked out? Especially important is to be aware of the issues that were problematic in your first marriage—whether they concerned sex, finances, arguing in destructive ways, spending time together, or extramarital affairs—and view them as "traps" to avoid in this relationship. Rather than ignoring the sensitive areas and hoping they won't recur, you need to disclose them to your new partner. If they start to cause difficulties you need to attend to them immediately. As the folk saying goes, "An ounce of prevention is worth a pound of cure." If you value this new marriage and want it to be successful both emotionally and sexually, you need to devote the time and psychological energy and communicate with your new partner in a respectful, cooperative manner.

BEING A WIDOWER

The death of a spouse is a severe trauma for the survivor, and it is normal to experience a variety of strong responses. In cases where the death of the wife is sudden, the husband's first—and natural—reaction will be to reject the situation as unreal, to feel that it can't be happening. Whether we realize it or not, a spouse fills a very large space in our lives. To have that presence removed without warning leaves a gulf we are incapable of comprehending at first. It can take months before the widower feels he is part of the world again. Especially for men under fifty, the idea of being a widower is a foreign one. For the older population, there are many more women who become widows than men who are widowers. Yet being a widower needs to be accepted and dealt with.

The next reaction is one of grief and depression. As the widower begins to take in the dimensions of his loss, the feelings of sadness seem overwhelming. At times he may find himself crying uncontrollably or experiencing a breakdown of self-control, which he needs to accept as natural. Painful, often maudlin, feelings and regrets may disturb him. He may think about things he and his wife had planned to do together and now will never have the chance for. He may feel guilty for not being more attentive or generous, for not buying her gifts she desired or taking her places she always wanted to go. He may even feel guilty simply because he is the survivor and can continue to live and enjoy things while the wife is deprived of life. Anger is not an uncommon reaction at this time. Many widowers feel furious at their wives for abandoning them, for leaving them alone—an irrational but natural feeling that the widowed man should try to accept. Feeling angry with a dead spouse does not mean you hated her; it is simply a sign of how important she was to you and how hard it is for you to reconcile yourself to her loss and the need for you to reestablish your own life. Anger is part of the grieving process.

Practical Issues Facing the Widower

Marriage involves not only emotional ties but practical considerations as well, and many of the feelings a widowed man experiences are connected with his sense of being overwhelmed with the responsibilities that are suddenly his alone. This is especially true when there are children to take care of. It is quite common for a widower to feel that it is unfair that he must suddenly do all the things he and his wife once shared, especially caring for the children's physical and emotional needs and running the household on a day-to-day basis. There is a temptation for the grief-stricken man to shut these responsibilities out by drinking heavily or by simply ignoring them. It is important for him to begin to take things in hand at this point, to recognize the problems that exist and face them head-on rather than trying to avoid them. It is not that he is not entitled to his grief, but rather that in the midst of grief he must deal with his present reality, which includes his responsibilities to his children. He must begin to look forward to the future and the rebuilding of his life.

Often the widowed man will find it impossible to take the full responsibility for home and family upon himself. It is a good idea for him to find a female friend or relative who he feels close to and comfortable with to help him manage things. Having someone who is familiar with the running of a household will make it much easier for the widower to begin living on his own. He should not reject help when offered on the grounds that he would prefer to be self-sufficient. It is not a sign of weakness to accept help while trying to adjust to the absence of a spouse. You are not seeking to establish a dependency on someone else but to use the support of others to help you act in a responsible way for yourself and your children. It is a sign of your commitment to reorganizing your life for the future.

It is very helpful if the widowed man has someone with whom he can share his strong and complex feelings of guilt, sadness, and anger. A friend, relative, minister, or family doctor often fulfills such a role. The widower might also consider seeking a professional counselor or psychologist who can help him to talk about, understand, and integrate his feelings. Whether he seeks out a professional or nonprofessional, there is no doubt that a newly widowed man needs somebody who can be a caring listener. Feelings produced by the death of a spouse—or by divorce, for that matter—if they are not allowed to come out, nearly always prove disruptive, and may prevent a man from making the transition to a successful single life.

If your wife died of a long, drawn-out disease such as cancer, accepting the fact of her death was certainly one of the most difficult tasks imaginable. Yet, it allowed you and your wife to prepare for her death. It was better for you and your dying spouse to deal with reality than to try to keep up a false front and pretend that everything was all right. A dying person needs closeness and support to help her accept what is happening. Attempting to maintain the pretense that all is well, that she will eventually recover, has the effect of isolating her in an envelope of unreality, of denying her the chance of expressing her true thoughts and feelings. By being dishonest to the dying spouse, however good his intentions, the survivor makes it harder on himself. Not only must he bear the strain of keeping up a pretense, but he makes it impossible to go through the psychological process of confronting death with the dying person. Thus, when death finally occurs, he is unprepared for the devastating effects of the loss.

SEXUAL ISSUES

What happens sexually during the wife's extended period of illness? The husband is likely to experience normal sexual desires. The first point to be made is that feeling the need for sex when his wife is terminally ill is not something a man should be dismayed about. Sexual desire is a basic and natural part of being alive. The question is in what ways can the couple integrate affectionate and sexual needs with the reality of the partner's dying.

Sexual relations between husband and wife can continue for as long as it is comfortable for both. If the wife's illness makes it impossible for her to engage in intercourse, the couple can continue to experience enjoyable sexual interactions through the use of other pleasuring techniques, from stroking and massaging to the use of manual or oral stimulation to orgasm. There is nothing "perverse" or offensive about continuing sexual relations when one spouse is dying. Indeed, a primary need of dying people is not to be rejected, ignored, or denied, but to feel that they are still cared about and worthwhile. One of the chief ways of affirming someone's worth is through tenderness, of which sexuality is an important expression, although certainly not the only one.

Sometimes sexual relations with the dying spouse may be limited or inappropriate, and in the latter stages of illness, sex may be unwanted or not possible. In such instances, masturbation can serve as an excellent sexual outlet for the man. He should not feel childish or selfish for engaging in masturbation, but look upon it as a sensible way for him to satisfy his very human needs within the confines of the situation. Another possibility, of course, is for the husband to seek sexual relations outside the marriage. Some couples have an implicit understanding that it is all right for the husband to become sexually involved with other women. Careful thought should be given, however, before going through with such a step. Since sexual relations often lead to feelings of emotional closeness with the partner, the husband might find that a sexual liaison with another woman would interfere with the closeness he wants to have with his spouse during her last months. Ultimately, it is a matter of weighing the alternatives involved—something each man must decide for himself according to his own circumstances and value system.

Once the death of the spouse has occurred, the widower faces a different set of sexual issues. Although he has lost his usual sex partner, he probably has not lost his sexual interest. Again, it is very important that the widower be aware that his sexual needs are quite normal and can be a source of pleasure to him. It is part of the life-affirming process. He shouldn't be embarrassed or ashamed of having sexual feelings, but view his continuing interest in sex as something positive, an indication of his will to survive and to continue leading an active and fulfilling life.

He may go through a period of exploration and experimentation in order to determine the best way, given his present needs and feelings, of expressing himself sexually. While some men find that they are at a point in their lives where sex is not very important to them, many more will wish to find a way of integrating sexual activity into their lives. There are several options available to them. For many widowers, masturbation is a helpful and enjoyable way to relieve sexual tensions. Masturbation is not abnormal or harmful, at this or at any other time, and it may be very beneficial and appropriate in situations where the widowered man is not ready to start a relationship. The widower should also be able, without feeling guilty, to think about and try out a variety of sexual and life patterns until he finds one that suits his needs and values. For example, he might seek out another partner for marriage; he might want a stable partner for sex and companionship without marriage; or he might wish to have a variety of briefer, less intense sexual relationships. Frequenting massage parlors or prostitutes may also be a sexual choice for the widowed or divorced man, although the need for intimacy and affection is less likely to be satisfied in this way.

One major problem widowers encounter is the feeling that if they become sexually involved with another woman they are being unfaithful to their dead wives. What the widower needs to realize is that it will not bring back his spouse if he deprives himself of emotional and sexual satisfaction; it will merely make his own life more unhappy and difficult. He owes it to himself to gain as much happiness as he can after the death of his spouse—most wives who really care for their husbands would not want it any other way—and a sexual relationship can be an important source of happiness. The fact that he has sex with other women does not mean that he did not love his wife; it simply means that he is a healthy male who chooses to continue with his life despite his loss.

THE WIDOWER'S SYNDROME

When he does find a new sex partner, however, the widower might find that he is a little out of practice romantically. Sex is a natural physiological response, but making love is a skill. Just as you do not play tennis or piano very well after several months or years away from it, when you resume sexual activity with a partner after a period of abstinence you will probably feel awkward and need time to regain your comfort and confidence. Anxiety, guilt, and other such feelings may intrude in these early experiences, causing such problems as erectile difficulty, rapid ejaculation, or ejaculatory inhibition. These difficulties are not unusual under the circumstances, and the man need not overreact or be discouraged. Through practice, he can become comfortable as a sexual partner again, and sexual functioning will return. If the sexual problems continue for more than six months, he might want to consult a sex therapist.

As he forms a new emotional and sexual attachment, the widower should avoid making comparisons between his new partner and his former wife. Experiences with a new partner, both sexual and otherwise, are likely to be very different from those with the previous spouse, and comparisons between them are not apt to do anyone very much good. Idealizing the dead wife can put pressure on the new partner and may cause her to feel discouraged and unloved. On the other hand, if the widower sees the new partner as superior, it may lead to feelings of guilt on his part. A happier course is for the man to refrain as far as possible from making comparisons and to deal with the new relationship on its own.

CLOSING THOUGHTS

Each widowed or divorced man faces issues that are unique to his special circumstances. I have attempted to deal with some of the most important problems in terms of male sexuality. Being widowered or divorced is difficult, an experience that causes pain, anguish, depression, and self-doubt. However rationally we deal with an experience of this kind, we cannot hope to escape entirely from its negative effects. However, by keeping in mind our basic worth as men and as human beings, by remaining positive about ourselves and affirming our right to happiness and fulfillment, we can recover from the loss and reorganize our lives. By affirming our sexuality and expressing our sexual feelings in a healthy way, we affirm ourselves as people. The single-again man needs to be aware that he has a number of alternatives, and needs to choose what is in his best interest.

22
"WITHIN THE NORMAL RANGE"
—UNDERSTANDING
MALE HOMOSEXUALITY

Before the last decade, books on sex treated homosexuality, if they dealt with it at all, primarily as a problem to be solved. It was assumed that the homosexual was abnormal, that something had gone wrong in his development, causing him to prefer a type of sexual expression that was unnatural and perverted, and that all homosexuals were unhappy and desperately lonely. Homosexuality was thought of as a sickness, and, like any sickness, it was considered to have an etiology (that is, specific cause) and a cure. The only trouble was that no one seemed to be able to identify very convincingly either the cause or the cure.

There has been a major change in attitudes and scientific knowledge about homosexuality in the past decade. Along with the liberalization of our attitudes toward sexuality in general, there has been an active gay movement (much like the movements of other minority groups) to demand the respect and equality that has been denied homosexuals. Many prominent people have openly declared their homosexual orientation, and great numbers of other individuals have proudly "come out of the closet." Phrases such as "gay pride" and "gay is good" have become commonplace. Meanwhile, recent findings by psychologists and other researchers have cast doubt on most of the assumptions the straight world has so smugly held about homosexuality. This research indicates that homosexuality is in no sense a disease but rather a normal variant of human sexual expression, no less "natural" or "healthy" than any other form of sexuality.

HOMOSEXUALITY AS A NORMAL VARIANT

The only sense in which homosexuality is "abnormal" is in the context of the values that are held by people of a particular society. Societies approve of certain patterns of behavior and disapprove of others. What is normal and desirable in one society may be abnormal and undesirable in another. Although homosexuality has existed in all times and in all cultures, the attitudes of different societies toward it have varied widely. In some instances it has been accepted as normal behavior (as, for instance, in ancient Greece); in other instances it has been condemned as sinful, perverse, and punishable by death (as in fundamentalist Iran). But homosexuality has remained constant— nothing more nor less than a powerful, emotional, and sexual preference for sexual partners of the same sex as oneself. Whether this preference is considered an abomination or a personal right has depended upon the values and attitudes of the people doing the judging.

In the United States, the laws and attitudes toward homosexuality are in a stage of reevaluation and change. The increasing strength and visibility of the gay movement and the more liberal general attitudes toward sexuality lend impetus to this newer and more accepting view of homosexuality. However, there are still a bewildering number of misconceptions, superstitions, and glaringly myth-based notions about homosexuality, even among the most sophisticated strata of the population. With the growing strength of fundamentalist religious groups and the fears raised by the disease AIDS, there has been a backlash of prejudice against homosexuality. This chapter will attempt to dispel these mistaken ideas, specifically with respect to male homosexuality, by exploring the subject in factual and nonbiased a manner as possible.

DATA ABOUT HOMOSEXUALITY

One widely held, but erroneous, notion is that people must be either exclusively heterosexual or exclusively homosexual. Alfred Kinsey made the point, based on numerous case histories, that homosexuality and heterosexuality can be envisioned as falling along a continuum, rather than being an either-or proposition. He found that the sex histories of many men revealed both heterosexual and homosexual feelings and experiences. For example, a man might have homosexual experiences during adolescence and become a practicing heterosexual as an adult. Another man, who has most of his sexual relationships with other males, might occasionally become aroused by a woman and have intercourse with her.

Approximately 75 percent of men have had at least one fantasy, thought, or feeling about another male that caused them to become aroused, usually occurring during adolescence or early adulthood. It is estimated that one out of every three men has at least one homosexual experience leading to orgasm sometime in his life, again usually in adolescence or early adulthood. About one in ten has been predominantly homosexual in his sexual expression for at least a year in his life. About 6 to 8 percent of males are essentially homosexual in their orientation. These facts are particularly important for heterosexual men who mistakenly believe that their sexual orientation must be pure and untainted and that if they have homosexual thoughts or an isolated homosexual experience this makes them "latent homosexuals." The much overused term *latent homosexuality* is neither very accurate nor useful. It serves to make men afraid and to reinforce antihomosexual feelings. This is the basis of the homophobia that is so rampant in our culture. Males are so afraid of their homosexual thoughts, feelings, fantasies, and/or experiences that they are very angry and belittling of homosexuals in order to combat any hint of "latent homosexuality" in themselves.

HOMOSEXUALITY IS NOT A MENTAL ILLNESS

Another common misconception is that homosexuality is a form of mental illness, a notion that is firmly entrenched in the public consciousness. Many people regard it as a matter of common sense that anyone who prefers partners of the same sex to partners of the opposite sex must be "sick" and in need of psychiatric help. True, many books and articles have been written by psychiatrists maintaining this point of view. But these writings are based on theorizing rather than factual evidence, and the case studies cited are drawn from the ranks of each psychiatrist's own patients—clearly a biased sample.

There is a good deal of solid scientific evidence to indicate that homosexuals, as a group, do not show any more pathology than heterosexuals. The family pressures and the societal and economic discrimination homosexuals have to deal with do add considerably more stress to their lives. In acknowledgment of such evidence and in response to pressure from the gay movement, both the American Psychological Association and the American Psychiatric Association have taken as their official position that homosexuality is not deviant behavior and is within the normal range of human sexual expression. This view of homosexuality has been accepted by most sex researchers and sex educators, including Masters and Johnson and the Kinsey Institute. For some men a homosexual orientation is the healthiest, most optimal life-style.

Homosexuality is best viewed as an emotional and sexual commitment to a person of the same sex rather than as an illness or a social problem. As long as homosexuality (or any other form of sexual activity, for that matter) is freely agreed upon by both partners, is performed in private, is not coercive, is not compulsive, does not cause physical injury, does not involve children, and is not used to inflict guilt or punishment on oneself or one's partner, it is within the range of normal and acceptable sexual behavior. This is not to say that homosexuality is in any way better than heterosexuality or that everyone should try it. What I am saying is that homosexuality needs to be accepted as a valid sexual orientation. It would be as equally erroneous to hold homosexuality as a sexual norm as it is to denigrate it as an inferior or unacceptable form of sexual expression.

PREJUDICE AGAINST GAYS

Many people believe that homosexual men can be identified by certain physical characteristics or peculiarities of dress and behavior. Some people congratulate themselves that their ability to identify homosexuals shows perceptiveness or sophistication, but in reality it is more likely to be a sign of prejudice similar to that of the anti-Semite who is convinced that he can "always spot a Jew." Actually, most homosexuals cannot be identified by outward signs. Most gay have no wish to stand out, and consequently keep a rather low profile looking, acting, and dressing as do other males in our culture. Nor is it true that homosexuals are to be found exclusively in certain characteristic occupations such as interior decorating or hairdressing. There are homosexuals in every field of endeavor, including stevedores, business executives, machinists, doctors, truck drivers, and college professors. Some homosexuals, of course, do dress and act in a flamboyantly effeminate manner, but they are in the minority and are often looked down upon and avoided by other gays who have no desire to flaunt their sexuality.

Despite the recent liberalization of attitudes, society continues to be hostile to gays. Homosexuality is still accepted as grounds for discharging a man from the armed forces, and in spite of a movement among the clergy to incorporate homosexuals into the religious community, the Roman Catholic Church continues to regard homosexuality as a perversion. Moreover, the attitude of most people toward homosexuality is still a poor one, ranging from disapproval to outright disgust. What are the reasons for this widespread and persistent antagonism?

It has to do with the notion that homosexuality is on the upswing and that unless it is kept down by force it will threaten the integrity of the family unit and the structure of society as a whole. There is no basis for this fear. Research indicates that there has been no change in the percentage of men who adopt a homosexual orientation. Homosexuality has become more visible because more and more individuals have openly declared themselves, but homosexuality does not pose a threat to the family unit. The great majority of males have been and will continue to be heterosexual; they will marry and produce more than enough children to ensure the perpetuation of society.

Fear of AIDs is the newest reason to excuse antihomosexual prejudices. Although AIDS is a very serious public health problem and of major concern to homosexual men, it is neither a homosexual nor a heterosexual disease, but rather a disease spread primarily by men.

Another reason many people fear homosexuality is that they are convinced that most homosexuals are child molesters. The homosexual who goes about seducing impressionable young boys is a figure of fear for many an anxious parent. Actually, it is an established fact that the majority of sex abusers of children are heterosexuals preying on young girls. Although there is a genuine problem of sexual abuse of male children, the men who do this constitute a very small minority of homosexuals.

A related, but more subtle fear, is that the increased acceptance of homosexuality will cause the male role to become less clearly defined, and this in turn will make it more likely for young boys to become homosexual. Many people are particularly opposed to homosexuals as teachers because of the fear that they might steer a young boy toward homosexuality at the point of his life when he is most impressionable and his sexual identity is in the process of formation. However, the data argue that these concerns, too, are largely groundless. Increased awareness and toleration does not lead to increased homosexuality.

Perhaps the most significant reason heterosexual men are hostile to homosexuals has to do with an apprehension that their own heterosexual orientation is somehow ambiguous or fraudulent, which is the basis for homophobia. Heterosexual men are afraid of being ''contaminated'' by contact with homosexuals. The heterosexual feels threatened because he fears that there is a homosexual part of him that the gay male might recognize and make a play for. This misapprehension is responsible for most cases of overreaction on the part of heterosexual men to sexual overtures by gays. The heterosexual feels that he has to protect his manhood from imagined contamination by reacting rudely, threateningly, or even by beating up the homosexual. Even if not approached, straight males will harass gay men on the street to show how ''macho'' they are. A man who is secure with his heterosexual orientation, however, feels no need to react in this way. He recognizes the invitation of the gay man for what it is—a mistake, a misdirected attempt to attract a sexual partner— and he responds simply by ignoring it or saying straightforwardly and assertively that he is not interested in a homosexual encounter.

Heterosexuals are particularly threatened by gay men because of the subtle indoctrination men in our society receive against excessive physical contact between males. We learn early that male contact should be strictly limited (for example, to competitive sports, a slap on the back, or a handshake). Even in father-son relationships, touching, playful roughhousing, and hugging usually comes to a halt as the boy grows older. Supposedly this restraint is in the interests of maintaining the social ideal of being "male." In contrast to this process of achieving "male identity," women are given freer reign to express themselves physically and emotionally. The demonstration of affection between women is generally accepted and does not seem to arouse fears that it will promote lesbianism or undermine "female identity." The one who loses to this irrational fear is the heterosexual man who would benefit from exchanging an affectionate hug with his best friend or child.

CAUSES OF HOMOSEXUALITY

Although many theories have been put forward to explain why certain individuals become homosexuals, the question remains largely unanswered. People ask "What went wrong to cause homosexuality?" Such an approach implies a biased and unscientific view, since it assumes that homosexuality necessarily involves a psychological or physical malfunction of some kind. A popular psychiatric theory suggests that homosexuals are the products of homes in which there is a dominant and seductive mother and a passive or absent father. Although the backgrounds of some homosexuals conform to this pattern, it is not true for the majority of gay men. Another leading theory is that homosexuality has some physiological basis such as a hormonal imbalance or a genetic predisposition. These factors might play a decisive roll for a small number of homosexual males. However, research has found that for the majority of homosexual men hormonal or genetic factors do not appear to play a major role. There are a number of other pseudoscientific theories bandied about with no research support.

A more constructive approach to the question of what causes homosexuality is to bear in mind that the decision about a sexual orientation, whether homosexual or heterosexual, is a complex phenomenon that is influenced by many interconnected factors—childbearing practices, the nature of peer interactions, sex education (or the lack thereof), ways of dealing with affection, body image, history of comfort and attraction, relationships between men and women, and early sexual experiences are possible influences on sexual orientation.

It is possible that a series of "pleasure events" in the presence of a member of the same sex might culminate in a later preference for male sex partners—a process analogous to what we hypothesize happens in the development of heterosexuality. The experiences of early orgasmic responses might be particularly important. The sexual fantasies males use during masturbation, especially if focused on one theme (sexual attraction to blue-eyed, blond men in their twenties, for example), might have a strong reinforcing effect on the development of sexual orientation. People learn to be sexual, and the nature of the learning determines whether one ultimately prefers opposite-sex or same-sex partners.

But regardless of what causes homosexuality, the most sensible and least prejudicial way of regarding sexual orientation is as a commitment to a way of life that is in accordance with one's emotional and sexual needs and desires. Whether a person decides on homosexuality, heterosexuality, or bisexuality, this commitment ought to be respected by other individuals, regardless of whether they share or approve of that particular orientation. It may be some time before such toleration is reached in our society, but when it comes it is sure to bring greater happiness and fulfillment than was ever achieved under the older prejudiced and repressive attitudes.

WHAT GAY MEN DO SEXUALLY

A great many misconceptions center around the methods used by gays to obtain sexual pleasure. It is assumed that the sexual practices of homosexuals include strange rituals and "kinky" and perverse acts. These notions exemplify the tendency of people to impute strange behavior to any group of which they have little direct knowledge. Although some gays do practice "exotic" sexual behavior, the percentage is probably no greater than that found among heterosexuals. Most of the sexual techniques used by gay couples are identical to those used by heterosexuals—a fact that underscores the absurdity of identifying any particular sexual technique as a specifically homosexual act. A homosexual interaction is defined by the fact that two same-sex people are involved, not by the nature of the technique employed. Thus, as we have seen, oral-genital contact between a man and a woman is not an indication of latent homosexual tendencies. Oral-genital contact is heterosexual if opposite-sex partners are involved and homosexual if same-sex partners are involved.

Fellatio is a form of sexual behavior commonly enjoyed by homosexual men. Fellatio might be mutual ("69 position"), or it might be performed by one partner at a time. It might be used solely as a sexual-arousal technique, or it might be carried to orgasm. Anal intercourse is another sexual technique engaged in by some gays and also tried by one out of seven heterosexual couples. Contrary to popular thinking, it is not the rule among homosexuals practicing anal intercourse for one partner to assume the female role and the other the male. It is more common to alternate in assuming the receptive and penetrative positions. However, since the AIDS epidemic, anal intercourse is being actively discouraged unless a condom is used and/or the couple is monogamous and both have been tested for the AIDS virus. Other forms of sexual expression used by gays include mutual manual stimulation, self-stimulation with partner present, frontage (mutual rubbing of the penis against the partner's body), and interfemoral intercourse (thrusting the penis between the partner's legs).

It is important to note that all of these activities can be and are engaged in by heterosexual as well as homosexual couples. (In fact, the only activity exclusive to heterosexuals is penis-vagina intercourse.) Homosexuals use these techniques with as much variation and imagination (or lack of it) as do heterosexuals. Kissing, caressing, and other pleasuring activities that form a part of heterosexual lovemaking are commonly incorporated into gay encounters as well.

Of course, some sex between gays—such as anonymous sexual encounters in men's toilets or at all-male public baths—is devoid of affection and emotion. But then so are most encounters between heterosexual men and prostitutes. These sexual experiences do not promote physical or mental health. This behavior has been reduced in frequency because it is not "safe sex," and if engaged in, condoms should be used and there should be no exchange of semen. The men who limit their homosexual encounters to brief, impersonal meetings are often those who are attempting to maintain a heterosexual facade and to satisfy their preference for male sexual contact on the sly.

The anonymity and lack of warmth may be blamed partially on the repressive intolerance of heterosexual society.

Homosexuals need and seek out closeness and intimacy in relationships. While a particular homosexual man has dominant sexual preferences, he is not likely to be inflexible and to engage in stereotyped and rigid patterns of sexual behavior. Like his heterosexual counterpart, he feels the need for spontaneity and variety and for greater sensual and emotional satisfaction in his sexual encounters.

GAY LIFE-STYLES

Life-styles among gays are diversified—a fact that runs counter to the idea that the majority of homosexuals are overconcerned with making sexual contacts to the exclusion of other life experiences. Many men succeed in integrating their homosexuality into their lives, engage in productive occupations, have a multitude of social and cultural interests, and establish satisfying friendships, as well as a romantic and sexual union with a lover. Because of the stigma attached to homosexuality in this culture, many homosexuals choose to express their sexual orientation clandestinely, admitting that they are gay only to other homosexuals and to intimate friends, and meanwhile representing themselves as straight to the rest of the world. Thus, they effectively lead two separate lives, sustain two independent identities. The psychological stress of such a life-style can be damaging. They are not yet able or willing to join the growing movement of gays who are open, vocal, and direct in affirming their sexual orientation, who proclaim that homosexuality is not a second-rate human condition and need not involve shame, guilt, or an apologetic attitude toward the rest of society.

Like any minority group, homosexuals place a high value on social institutions that allow them to enjoy the company of others who share their own preferences and problems. Hence, the continuing popularity of gay bars. Essentially, the gay bar serves the same purpose for homosexuals as the singles cocktail lounge serves for heterosexuals. Not all gay men enjoy these bars; some, in fact, avoid them, preferring other kinds of social activities such as small dinner parties or team sports. "Cruising" (seeking out sexual contacts) involves walking or driving around in areas that have a heavy concentration of other gays seeking sexual liaisons. Cruising—whether it occurs in a bar, party, class, or at an intersection—involves a subtle and complex system of nonverbal cues not unlike the seductive behavior common among heterosexually oriented people. In some areas, male prostitution (or "hustling") may also occur.

Sexual relationships between homosexual men are less permanent than heterosexual relationships or relationships between lesbians. To a certain extent, however, this impermanence can be attributed to the corrosive effect of society's negative attitude toward male homosexual attachments. Long-term relationships between heterosexual couples are encouraged in all kinds of ways by society, particularly when they are formalized by marriage and involve children. Female homosexuality, while not approved by society, arouses less hostility. Women are traditionally allowed to be more physically expressive with one another; unmarried women are almost expected to live together as roommates. Hence, a lesbian couple can maintain a relationship without attracting as much attention as a male homosexual couple.

Nevertheless, many gay men establish relationships that last five, ten, or twenty years, and even longer. Some gay couples have, in fact, sought to legitimize their relationships as formal marriages, insisting that to deny them the same rights and advantages that are accorded to heterosexual couples constitutes blatant discrimination. There is growing support for more permanent and monogamous gay relationships.

Gays have attempted to organize in other ways. The Gay Activist Alliance, along with other advocacy groups, is working for an end to discrimination against homosexuals in hiring practices, living arrangements, and other social situations. Gay religious groups are attempting to bring about the acceptance of homosexuals within the religious establishment. There are "Dignity" groups, masses for gay Catholics, and gay community churches. Such organizers underscore the fact that gays are human beings whose choice of sexual orientation and life-style is a legitimate one that should in no way preclude them from enjoying the same freedom and privileges accorded to other people. "Problem-centered" groups and services such as "Gay Alcoholics Anonymous," gay switchboards, and gay clinics have been established to deal with specific difficulties faced by homosexuals. Support groups for men with AIDS are a recent and very worthwhile phenomenon.

DECISION MAKING ABOUT SEXUAL ORIENTATION

As we observed at the beginning of this chapter, sexual orientation falls along a continuum, with some men experiencing arousal in both homosexual and heterosexual interactions. It might seem that those men who have tendencies in both directions ought to be able to express themselves as homosexuals and as heterosexuals, according to the circumstances. However, such an adjustment is rarely possible. The majority of individuals find it quite difficult to function as active bisexuals. Straddling both worlds places serious social and psychological stresses on the individual that are very difficult to sustain. Thus, most men who feel strongly drawn toward homosexuality must make a conscious decision at some point to either actively accept their homosexual orientation or attempt to reinforce their potential for functioning as a heterosexual.

Such a commitment must ultimately rest with the individual himself based on what he feels would lead to the greatest pleasure, fulfillment, and happiness for him. His decision should not be based on what others want for him, whether those others happen to be parents, a wife, his religion, an employer, or society at large. While it is true that those who are closest to a person feel that they want what is best for him, their very emotional involvement makes them unable to provide unbiased and nonjudgmental advice. It is the individual himself who must live with the decision, so it is he who must assume the responsibility for making it.

Nor is it advisable for a man to procrastinate when making a decision about his sexual orientation. Difficult as life may be for a homosexual in certain instances, there are few things more painful for a man than to go through the motions of heterosexual existence while fighting against the belief that his true emotional and sexual needs would be better fulfilled as a homosexual. One of the most common mistakes is to marry as an attempt to avoid the issue. These marriages often turn out to be shams where the man is leading a double life. One of the most difficult situations is that of the man who, fearing to confront his homosexual orientation, chooses to deny his sexual needs altogether and makes no sexual contacts with people of either sex. Such a person condemns himself to living a shadow existence in both worlds while enjoying the advantages of neither.

We are all sexual beings whether we admit it or not, and we have a right to some form of sexual and emotional expression. To deny this fact is to shut off one of the major sources of happiness in your life—but that, too, is an individual decision. For a man making the commitment to a sexual orientation, professional guidance can be invaluable. A professional therapist, if he is truly qualified to help in these situations, will not attempt to force a particular decision on the client, but rather will help him discover what his real needs are and then to assist him in planning a course of action designed to realize them. This professional may be a psychologist, a minister, a psychiatric social worker, a psychiatrist, or an individual working for a gay counseling service. His effectiveness will depend less on his professional qualifications than on his commitment to helping the client achieve a personally satisfying decision. In my own practice I have counseled quite a number of men seeking help in committing to a sexual orientation, and in each case my guiding principle has been that the needs and desires of the client come first. A solution to the issue (or any other sexual problem) that is imposed from without is no solution at all.

Tom

Tom was a nineteen-year-old college student who had been a practicing homosexual since he was thirteen. The summer before, Tom's parents found out about his homosexual activities and insisted that he seek professional therapy. He presented himself as a reluctant client, making it clear that he was coming to a therapist under duress and that he expected me to share his parents' disapproving attitude. My first task was to make clear that I viewed homosexuality as a legitimate sexual alternative and that it was not my intention to force him to change. We decided that we would spend three sessions reviewing his sexual development and preferences and then determine a plan of action. Tom decided that a homosexual orientation would be better for him since his sexual experiences, masturbatory fantasies, and emotional and sexual preferences all pointed toward an overwhelming attraction for other men. We then focused on how to describe this to his parents in a way they could accept without blaming themselves for the fact that Tom was committed to homosexuality. Tom realized that it would be unrealistic to expect them to be enthusiastic about his decision, at least at first, and that simple acceptance was the most he could hope for. This turned out to be the right approach; Tom's parents eventually became reconciled to his homosexuality, an adjustment that contributed greatly toward relieving the tension that had developed in the family. It allowed Tom to focus on the crucial issue—how he could be successful as a gay person—personally, sexually, emotionally, and in his career. This commitment to leading a successful and satisfying life is an integral part of accepting one's homosexuality.

George

Another client, George, was a twenty-one-year-old man who felt very ambivalent about his sexual orientation. Since the age of fourteen, he had felt admiration and attraction for athletic and virile men. Convinced that he had a small penis, he was aroused by the thought of men with large organs. Although George masturbated frequently to a variety of homosexual, heterosexual, bisexual, and group-sexual fantasies, his sexual experiences with other people were limited. He had had two successful homosexual experiences in which he was fellated to orgasm, and one unsuccessful heterosexual intercourse experience in which he ejaculated before he could insert his penis into the woman's vagina. George wanted to see me to discuss his confused sexual feelings. I began by telling him that the decision to be straight or gay was ultimately his. After four or five sessions in which we explored his sexual experiences, feelings, values, and fantasies, George decided that it would be better for him to commit to a heterosexual orientation. We then engaged in a systematic program to increase his heterosexual arousal and skills and to decrease his homosexual desires and feelings. This relearning process proved successful, and George went on to function happily as a heterosexual. He was able to experience both sexual arousal with women and enjoy emotional intimacy in a way he could not with males.

A RATIONAL VIEW OF HOMOSEXUALITY

For the sake of homosexuals and heterosexuals alike, it would be best if society could adopt the basic principle that serves as a guide for responsible therapists: sexual orientation is a matter the individual himself must be free to decide in his own best interest. Those committing to a homosexual orientation should be given as much respect as those who make the heterosexual decision. Homosexuality should be looked upon as a truly alternative way of life, not a second-rate one. We must remember that a homosexual is above all else a human being, and we should emphasize the positive aspects of his humanness rather than stigmatize him with the label of deviant. Contrary to what you may have heard there is such a thing as a successful gay person. I have met quite a few of them. Whether we will be meeting more of them in the future depends at least in part on the attitude that straights decide to adopt. The most important thing, however, is the self-acceptance of the gay person himself and his commitment to be successful in his own emotional and sexual life.

23

SEXUALLY TRANSMITTED DISEASES—STDS

STDs, sexually transmitted diseases, were previously called VDs—veneral diseases. It's a depressing reality that you can get a disease from making love. And yet, STDs are a very real concern. They are, in fact, the most prevalent infectious diseases next to the common cold. To leave them out of a discussion of sexuality would be unrealistic. A major premise of this book is that a person must take responsibility for his behavior and accept the consequences of it whether pleasant or unpleasant. STDs can be an unfortunate consequence of sex, and thus they are an eventuality that may have to be dealt with by anyone who engages in sex.

It is important to keep one distinction firmly in mind. You don't get an STD because you have sex. It isn't a judgment, a punishment, a bacterial sword of Damocles waiting to fall on the sexual transgressor. Rather, you contract an STD through sex contact, which is a very different thing. The idea that an STD is one of the penalties of sex has long been used by moralists for the suppression of sexual activity. It is an old and tenacious fallacy, akin to the medical notion that plagues came about as a direct result of the sinful behavior of the populace. There has been a recent resurgence of this type of thinking because of our experiences with AIDS and herpes, two STDs that are not curable. The fact that such ideas gain widespread acceptance attests to the capacity of human beings to feel irrational guilt rather than to the idea's validity. The medieval plagues were caused not by sin but by poor sanitation. Similarly, the current epidemic of STDs is not a punishment we have brought down upon ourselves through increased sexuality, but the result of ignorance and lack of sexual responsibility. It is the consequence of our failure to face a problem squarely, to plan our sexual activities, and to take responsibility for our sexual behavior.

Avoiding sex because it can give you an STD is not the answer. After all, you can contract influenza by breathing in viruses that have been exhaled by an infected person, and you can catch hepatitis by eating contaminated food—hardly valid reasons for either avoiding the company of other human beings or refusing to take in nourishment. The situation with STDs is similar. The answer is not to avoid sex, but to be aware of the ways of preventing, detecting, and treating STDs so that this medical problem does not interfere with your life and sexual functioning.

DATA ABOUT STDS

Connected with the idea that STDs are a punishment for sexual activity is the notion that only morally "degenerate" and "dirty" people contract STDs. It is common for people to think that an STD "can't happen to me," that it is contracted only by a vaguely defined group of people who are morally and socially inferior to oneself. When a person who thinks in these term contracts an STD, his reaction is one of intense surprise and shame: "This can't be happening to me—not me!" He feels that having an STD brands him as precisely one of those undesirable individuals he previously scorned. He may turn on the sex partner he suspects of having given him an STD and accuse her of being a "whore." Such an attitude makes little sense when one considers the extreme prevalence of STDs. In 1987, there were over one million reported cases of gonorrhea alone, and since most cases go unreported, it is estimated that the actual figure was more like two and a half million. In the face of such numbers, it becomes clear that STDs must be taken seriously by all of us.

If there is any group more prone to STDs than others, it is the young, for the highest incidence rate is found among individuals between the ages of fifteen and nineteen. But STDs attack people of all ages, races, religions, sexual orientations, and socioeconomic groups. If you think for a moment about the extent of the networks formed in our society through sexual contact, it will become obvious that there are very few people who are not potential STD victims. An STD is a medical disease, not a moral judgment or a sign of the kind of person you are.

How does one contract an STD? In order to answer this question, it is necessary to distinguish between the four most common and serious STDs: gonorrhea, herpes, chlamydia, and syphilis. Gonorrhea (also known as "clap," "dose," and "strain") is passed from person to person through genital contact. Heterosexual intercourse is not the only way the disease is transmitted, however. It is also possible to contract gonorrhea through oral and anal sex. It follows that it can be transmitted through homosexual as well as heterosexual contacts, and, in fact, the recorded STD rate among homosexual males is considerably higher than among heterosexual males.

Herpes is a viral infection that once contracted remains in the person's body, although usually latent. Herpes can only be transmitted through direct genital contact when the person is in a herpes cycle (that is, contagious because there is an outbreak of herpes sores). Herpes is contracted by any contact with the herpes sores.

Chlamydia is an organism spread by sexual contact that infects the genital organs of both males and females. In males, the symptoms are a thin, clear discharge and mild pain on urination. Females are usually without symptoms. Unfortunately, it is fast becoming the most common STD in our country, partly because partners reinfect each other. It is essential that both partners be treated at the same time.

Syphilis (also known as "pox," "bad blood," and "syph") is transmitted by close, intimate contact that is usually, but not always, sexual. It is quite possible, for example, for syphilis to be transmitted by kissing if one of the partners has an infection or chancre in his or her mouth. The germs that cause both syphilis and gonorrhea die very quickly if they are not in a warm, moist environment. Thus, contrary to popular notions, it is impossible to catch an STD through contact with unsanitary toilet seats.

Statistics indicate that about one out of every three people in our society will contract an STD at some point in their lives.

Since it is impossible to be certain that you will never become a victim of an STD, it is a good idea to know how to recognize whether you have one or not. With the growing public hysteria about AIDS, the other STDs have been ignored as being unimportant. This is not true in terms of incidence, so let us begin by discussing the major STDs.

GONORRHEA

Gonorrhea is the very common STD (the cases of it outnumber syphilis by ten to one) and is passed from person to person through genital contact. Major symptoms in men are a burning sensation in the urethra during urination, and a heavy discharge of whitish or yellowish pus from the penis. These symptoms occur in most cases, but some males contract gonorrhea without developing any discernible symptoms. Untreated or improperly treated gonorrhea can result in kidney problems, bladder infections, blood poisoning, and even arthritis.

Gonorrhea is considerably more difficult to detect in women because they usually experience no symptoms, although some do feel pain while urinating and have a vaginal discharge. Untreated gonorrhea in women can lead to even more severe problems than in men, including pelvic inflammatory disease, sterility, and uterine infections. The incubation period for gonorrhea in both men and women is from two to ten days. The symptoms, if any, begin to appear after this period.

The only sure way to determine whether or not you have gonorrhea is to go for a test at a doctor's office or health clinic. The test used, a smear and culture, is the only definitive way of determining whether a person has the disease. A blood test, or VDRL, which is used to test for syphilis, will not reveal the presence of gonorrhea. It is a good idea, by the way, to specifically request a VDRL test in addition to a smear and culture, even if the symptoms you display point to gonorrhea rather than syphilis. It is quite possible to have both diseases at the same time. Fortunately, most gonorrhea can be easily cured by treatment with penicillin or by another antibiotic drug.

HERPES

Herpes can only be diagnose when there is an active outbreak of sores. When this occurs you can go to your general physician, urologist, or dermatologist, who will take a scraping from the sores, analyze it, and tell you whether or not it is herpes. If you do have herpes, you need to be an aware patient but not overreact. Although it is true that at present there is no cure for herpes, its effects are less severe than for gonorrhea and syphilis. Some people will have a single herpes outbreak and then the disease will remain dormant. A more typical pattern is for the herpes outbreaks to start off weeks or months apart, and then gradually decrease in frequency and intensity. It is crucial that the man be aware of his herpes cycle and refrain from any direct genital contact with the herpes sores during an outbreak (or during your partner's outbreak). Even if both people already have herpes this should be rigidly adhered to because of reinfection by additional herpes virus agents. The couple can engage in sexual stimulation during a herpes outbreak or one partner can stimulate the other, but great care must be taken to totally avoid all contact with herpes sores.

AIDS

The term AIDS (Acquired Immune Deficiency Syndrome) is enough to cause terror in not only men, but women as well, not only in the United States, but throughout the world. In fact, some mental health people talk about FAIDS (Fear of AIDS) syndrome. AIDS is a new disease, not diagnosed until about 1980, and needs to be taken seriously as a major public health threat, and as having the potential to become a worldwide epidemic. However, the current atmosphere of fear, stigma, and moralistic pandering to people's misconception by calling it God's revenge on homosexuals, or nature's way of containing sex, or God's punishment for sexual wickedness, is counterproductive.

Let us first examine the presently known scientific facts about AIDS from an objective perspective and then discuss how we can be responsible, practice safe sex, and take care of our sexual health. First, AIDS is a virus that is spread primarily through the mediums of blood and semen. Although it is present in other mediums—saliva, tears, sweat, etc.—at present it appears very unlikely that the disease will be transmitted in that way. Second, AIDS is not a disease of sexual orientation; it can be transmitted to both heterosexuals and homosexuals. Third, it appears that when it comes to sexual contact (as opposed to blood transmission, as when using contaminated needles) AIDS is a disease passed from males to females or males to males. In other words, it is principally males who transmit the disease. Transmission from female to male, although possible, appears extremely rare. Fourth, the carriers of AIDS are healthy men who have no symptoms and will not develop AIDS, but who remain infectious and are carriers indefinitely. Fifth, the means of transmission sexually is through semen entering the other person's body whether through vaginal, oral, or anal transmission.

The reason there have been so many cases of AIDS in the homosexual community is the number of sexual partners some gay men have (thus, the carrier infects many men) and the use of anal intercourse (which can break small blood vessels in the anal area, thus mixing blood and semen, which presents the greatest risk for AIDS transmission). Males who are passive in anal intercourse are the highest risk group for AIDS.

However, it is equally possible for a male who has the AIDS virus in his bloodstream to infect a female by semen entering her vagina, mouth, or anus. In some countries, AIDS is more common in the heterosexual than homosexual community.

Prevention of AIDS

Since there is no cure for AIDS at present, and it is a terminal disease, prevention is the obvious answer. There are three levels of prevention. The first is to limit your sexual activity to heterosexual sex. For the woman it is to limit her sexually activity to partners she knows only function heterosexually and do not use intravenous drugs. The second level is to be sure the person you are sexually active with is free from the AIDS antibodies. You need to have a direct, assertive conversation about STDs, and AIDS specifically, to determine if the person might be at risk for contracting the disease. If so, and you were to establish an ongoing relationship with the person, you could assertively request they take an AIDS test. There are clinics and some private doctors who allow you to take the test using a number or fictitious name (to insure your confidentiality) and to pay cash (so the transaction would not be recorded for health insurance purposes). The initial AIDS screening test is calibrated in such a way that it gives a high number of false positives. Thus, there are a number of people who do not carry the virus but test positive. If a positive result occurs, instead of panicking, the person should take the second test, which is more discriminating.

The third level of prevention is to practice safe sex. This means not allowing a person to ejaculate inside of you (orally or anally, and for women vaginally). The other safe sex procedure is for the male to wear a condom in vaginal, oral, and anal sex.

If a Person Tests Positive

A positive result on the more sophisticated AIDS screening test means that you have the AIDS antibodies in your bloodstream and that you will be a carrier all your life. It does not mean you will necessarily develop AIDS. In fact, the majority of carriers do not become infected with AIDS. You can protect your health and reduce the likelihood of developing AIDS by living an especially healthy life. This means good eating, sleeping, and exercising habits, not smoking or using drugs, and very moderate drinking. Consult with your physician about other steps you can take to protect your health and immune system.

Having a positive AIDS antibodies test means a dramatic change in your sexual expression. You will not be able to engage in any sexual activity that involves exchange of body fluids, that is, you cannot ejaculate inside anyone or have them ejaculate inside you. You can engage in sensual and sexual expression, but it needs to be limited; you can stimulate yourself or your partner can stimulate you to orgasm, but you can't utilize oral or intercourse sex. Since this is an area of medical and psychological uncertainty, I would urge you to seriously consider joining a support group for people who have tested positive. The group can provide emotional encouragement as well as correct information and practical suggestions.

AIDS is a very serious medical problem that needs to be addressed by both men and women, heterosexuals and homosexuals. The better informed you are about AIDS, the more you can objectively determine whether you are at risk and behave in a safe-sex, health-promoting manner. People governed by fears and panic do not take beneficial steps; people who value themselves and their sexuality will take appropriate steps to guard their health.

DEALING WITH AN STD RATIONALLY

An STD, because of its peculiar symptomatology, is frequently difficult to detect and, therefore, often goes untreated. However, the medical difficulties of treating the disease are insignificant compared with the psychological resistance that prevents the majority of its victims from dealing with it in a rational manner. Particular diseases affect our images as people in particular ways. Certain diseases are considered socially acceptable, while others are not. Thus, a person who has suffered a heart attack may feel affronted or despondent that his body has failed him, but it would probably not occur to him to hide the nature of his malady from others. However, most people feel intense shame when they find that they are suffering from an STD. They feel that the disease identifies them with the world of prostitutes, of seamy, lower-class characters slowing rotting away from the consequences of their immoral lives. So intense is this shame that many victims will not allow themselves to believe that they actually have an STD, even after the symptoms manifest themselves unmistakably. How could they have an STD when they are simply "not that sort of person"?

Because of this view of STDs, many people who contract them either avoid obtaining treatment or wait so long before seeing a doctor that complications occur that lead to permanent damage. Other victims may seek treatment in time, but go to great lengths to see that the matter is "hushed up." Unfortunately, many doctors are willing to cater to this anxiety. The law requires all STD cases to be reported to the health authorities. The information about sexual partners, embarrassing as it may be to divulge, is necessary so that those people who may have been exposed to infection can be notified, tested, and treated. Because the symptoms are not always noticeable, especially among women, it may be quite a while before the female realizes she has an STD. Meanwhile, the infection may spread from one person to another until dozens, perhaps hundreds, have been affected.

It is obvious that the microorganisms that cause the diseases have no interest in the social status of their victims. As far as STDs are concerned, we are all one big family, and it makes no more sense to be ashamed of catching an STD than it does to be ashamed of catching measles. Moreover, whatever shame may be connected with an STD should be more than outweighed by your sense of responsibility to your own well-being, to society in general, and especially to the people you choose as your sex partners. Responsibiltiy ought to be the keynote of all our sexual involvements.

In view of the ease with which most STDs can be cured once detected, there is no excuse for the fact that their occurrence has grown in our society to epidemic proportions. There have been public information and advertising campaigns aimed at providing accurate information concerning STDs. Free STD clinics have been set up that treat all patients confidentially, including those under legal age. Ways of recognizing, treating, and preventing STDs have been shown on TV and in magazines.

Despite all these efforts, however, the incidence of STDs is still on the increase. The shame connected with the diseases continues to be intense, and until steps are taken to correct this situation, irrational and self-defeating behavior will remain the rule. The public's attitude toward STDs resembles the syndrome of fear, denial, and embarrassment that until recently surrounded breast cancer and prevented women from being tested and seeking treatment. The turning point for breast cancer occurred in the 1970s, when, in rapid succession, Betty Ford and Happy Rockefeller announced they had breast cancer. The example set by these two public figures—the wives of the president and the vice president—encouraged women to learn more about breast cancer, to begin monthly breast self-exams, and to obtain periodic examination by a physician. As a result, there has been a dramatic increase in the detection of breast cancer in its early stages. It would be a great step toward bringing STD under control if comparable public figures were to perform a similar service with respect to these diseases. Considering their prevalence, there should not be any lack of opportunity, and the example of one or two courageous persons might be all that would be needed to bring about a wholesale change in the public's attitude toward STDs.

MALE RESPONSIBILITY TO INFORM PARTNERS

In a sense, we men are fortunate because the symptoms of STDs in men are more distinct, and the chances of detecting them in their early stages are much greater than in women, who usually have no symptoms. Reservations about seeking treatment are overcome by the obvious physical discomfort a man experiences when he has gonorrhea. Whatever a man's motivations in seeking treatment, though, the responsible and compassionate thing for him to do if he finds that he has gonorrhea or any other STD is to inform anyone with whom he has had intimate contact. By doing so, he may help his partner to detect an STD in its early stages and avoid the consequences of the later forms of the disease. The effects of untreated gonorrhea are particularly severe in women; moreover, since nine out of ten women exhibit no noticeable symptoms, the danger that significant damage will occur before the disease is identified is great.

The problem of how to tell a sex partner she should be tested and, if necessary, treated for an STD is complex, particularly if informing her of the facts involves revealing that you have had other sexual contacts she was unaware of. There is no "right" way to do this, but for the sake of your partner's health it is crucial that you convey the information to her. You can either take the responsibility yourself or have medical authorities contact her. The latter alternative is, of course, the less courageous one, but at least it gets the job done, and that is the main thing. Whichever way you choose, and whatever the possible consequences to the relationship, the only sensible course of action is to tell your partner, since the health hazards of untreated STDs are so great.

Ralph

The discovery of an STD can present difficult psychological problems in addition to the obvious medical ones. Ralph, a twenty-eight-year-old salesman, was engaged to be married, but still indulged in casual affairs while on sales trips away from home. Three months before the date set for the wedding, during one such trip, he had sex with a woman he met in a bar. He came home on a Friday and spent a sexually active weekend with his fiancée. Four days later, Ralph noticed a burning sensation in his penis during urination. Suspecting gonorrhea, he went to his physician for tests. The test results were positive, so the doctor treated Ralph with penicillin, but did not urge him to supply the names of recent sex partners. Thus, Ralph had to decide for himself what to tell his fiancée. For a day or two, he was tortured by doubts and indecision. Actually, he had no way of telling whether he had caught the STD from the woman he'd met in the bar or from his fiancée herself. If his fiancée was responsible, then this meant she had another sex partner, and despite his own infidelities, Ralph found this infuriating. But whether she had infected him or not, chances were that she now had the disease herself and would have to be told sooner or later. For several more days Ralph attempted, through indirect questioning, to determine whether she had had sexual relations with anyone besides himself. Finally, getting nowhere with these questions, he decided to tell her straight out. He did so, and she accepted the news far more calmly than he had anticipated. Ralph went with her to her gynecologist for a smear and culture, which were positive. The episode was not pleasant for either of them, but on the whole, Ralph's fiancée felt more reassured about Ralph's concern for her welfare than she felt hurt by his having had sex with another woman. The wedding took place on schedule.

PREVENTION

There are three primary methods of preventing STDs. The first is to only have sex with your partner or be very discriminating about the people you have sexual relations with. But since no particular class of people is immune from STDs, this method can never be totally successful. The second method is to use a condom when having sex, particularly with someone you do not know well. The third is to urinate and wash the genitals with soap before and after sexual contact.

A secondary method of dealing with the possibility of STD is to take steps to insure early detection. In addition to being alert to the onset of the physical symptoms, a man who is sexually active with a number of different partners should have a smear and culture as well as a VDRL test administered at least once a year and preferably every six months. These tests are not typically given as part of a regular physical examination, so it is necessary to request them specifically.

Throughout this book it is assumed that the best and most realistic criterion for judging if a particular sexual practice is acceptable or not is whether it is harmful in some way to either your partner or yourself. It is indisputable that you cannot do yourself good by harming others. An STD greatly enlarges the possibility of your harming others through sex or of being harmed by them. But basically, the ethics governing one's attitude toward STDs need not be any different from the ethics of sexuality in general. Behavior that is based on awareness, caring, compassion, and responsibility will serve you well.

EPILOGUE

We live in a time of rapidly changing attitudes and behaviors. Many of the ideas and values that were taken for granted as recently as ten years ago are no longer valid. Attitudes toward sexuality are among those that have undergone the greatest change. Men used to be very certain of their place in the world. They occupied the most important positions; they were the decision makers, the leaders. In the domestic realm, the man was supreme. "Every man is a king in his own household" went the slogan. This was particularly true of sexual relationships. Men were considered the ones who had a greater need for sex, who had a greater knowledge of sex, and who enjoyed sex more. They initiated sexual encounters when it pleased them to do so, and it was the woman's duty to follow their lead. Even the sexual position that enjoyed the greatest popularity—male on top—stressed the dominance of men over women.

Now all this is changing. There are holdouts, of course—both men and women who cling to the double standard, who want the old male-centered domestic and sexual monarchy to endure. These traditionalists are fighting a losing battle. Sexual equality is one of the building principles of today's world and will continue to be in the future. In business, politics, interpersonal relations, and in sex, women are demanding the autonomy that has for so long been denied them. The research evidence is clear—intellectually, behaviorally, emotionally, and sexually there are many more similarities than differences between men and women. Eventually, sexual equality will be an accomplished fact.

288

As men, I think we ought to rejoice that this is finally coming about. The double standard was never really in our interest anyway. It emphasized what was different in the sexual responses of men and women rather than what was similar. Under the double standard, we were led to believe that a man's only interest in sex was intercourse and orgasm—"getting your rocks off." Everything else was just frills. Women, on the other hand, were supposed to care primarily about gentle caresses, intimate emotions, lingering kisses—"romance and flowers." It was as if men and women were two entirely different species— each with its own sexual habits.

Today, however, with the decline of the double standard and the increase in scientific research into human sexual behavior and response, it is becoming increasingly clear that men and women have very similar sexual and emotional needs. Men are finding that gentleness, sensual awareness, and intimacy greatly enhance their sexual response. Women are finding that their need for direct genital stimulation, their capacity for orgasm, and their sexual desire are as great as men's. Some men find the idea of a woman who is as sexually active and responsive as themselves threatening. A far better attitude, however, would be to celebrate the fact that men and women, after so many years of alienation, have an opportunity to develop a respectful, cooperative, and satisfying emotional and sexual relationship. Having discovered that their sexual needs and desires are so similar, they can now collaborate on finding the best ways of fulfilling them.

I hope that this book will represent a step toward bringing about grater awareness, respect, and sexual expression for men and women. While many recent publications have been devoted to awakening women to the aspects of their sexuality that have for too long been ignored, there has been a paucity of similar works directed at men. My aim has been both to provide accurate information on male sexuality and to influence men to become more sensually aware, more responsible for their own sexuality, more able to communicate with their partner about sexual matters, more conscious of the part that sexuality plays throughout their lives, and more able to integrate their sexuality with their personal and emotional lives. Such changes may seem like a lot to ask for, and yet, there are few areas in which there are such powerful incentives for change.

It is in a man's—any man's—best interest to make the transition from sexual machine to sexual person. By doing so, he can increase not only his sexual pleasure but also his general level of satisfaction with himself, his spouse, his family, with life in general. It is time we realize what a positive element our sexuality can be and how we can use it to make our existence and our relationships more rewarding.

APPENDIX I
HOW TO FIND A THERAPIST

As I stated at the onset, this book is not meant to be a do-it-yourself therapy book. Many men are reluctant to consult a professional therapist, feeling that to do so is a sign of "craziness," inadequacy, or weakness. But I believe that it is actually a sign of psychological strength in that doing so means a man is able to accept the fact that there is a problem and to make a commitment to problem solving, positive change, and psychological and sexual growth.

The mental health field is a confusing one. There are many approaches to counseling and therapy, and a number of different types of professionals in the field. In sorting this out, your first concern should be to find someone who is professionally competent in the area of your problem. Psychotherapy encompasses various techniques, and it is offered by several different groups of professionals, including psychologists, psychiatrists, sex therapists, social workers, marriage therapists, and pastoral counselors. The particular label of the practitioner is of less importance than his or her competency in your special area of need.

In obtaining a referral for a therapist, one of the best resources is to call a local professional organization (psychological association, mental health association, or mental health clinic). Another method is to ask for a referral from a family physician, minister, or friends who might have some information on the therapist's areas of competence.

Many people have health insurance that provides coverage for mental health services, and thus can afford the services of a private practitioner. Those who do not have either the financial resources or the insurance could consider a city or county

291

mental health clinic or perhaps a university or medical school mental health outpatient clinic, which usually provides services on a sliding-fee scale (that is, the fee is based on your ability to pay).

In choosing a specific therapist, be assertive enough to ask about their credentials and areas of expertise as well as fees. A competent professional therapist will be open to discussing this with you. Be especially diligent in discussing credentials (university degrees, licensing) with people who call themselves personal counselors, marriage counselors, or sex counselors, since there are some poorly qualified persons (and some out-and-out quacks) working in any field.

If you have a problem that deals principally with marriage or family issues, you could write the American Association for Marriage and Family Therapy, 1717 K Street, NW, Washington, D.C. 20006, for a list of certified marriage and family therapists in your area. If you have a specific behavior problem, such as a phobia, lack of assertion, overeating, alcoholism, or sexual anxiety, you could write the Behavior Therapy and Research Society, c/o Eastern Pennsylvania Psychiatric Institute, Henry Avenue, Philadelphia, Pennsylvania 19129, for a list of certified behavior therapists in your area. If you are specifically interested in sex therapy, you could write the American Association of Sex Educators, Counselors, and Therapists at Suite 220, Eleven Dupont Circle, Washington, D.C. 20036, or call 202-462-1171, for a list of certified sex therapists in your area.

Do not hesitate to talk to two or three therapists before deciding on one with whom to work. You need to be aware of your degree of comfort with the therapist, whether you feel you can relate to him or her, and whether the therapist's assessment of the problem and approach to treatment make sense to you. However, once you begin therapy, give it a chance to be helpful. There are few "miracle cures," and change requires your commitment and is a gradual and often difficult process. It is not like going to a medical doctor, who might prescribe pills and tell you exactly what to do. The role of the therapist is that of an adviser or counselor rather than that of one who decides upon a change for you. Psychotherapy requires effort, but it can be well worth it as measured by changed attitudes, feelings and behavior, and making your life more functional and pleasurable.

APPENDIX II
SUGGESTED READING

Andry, Andrew, and Schepp, Steve. *How Babies Are Made*. Boston: Little, Brown & Co., 1984.

Barbach, Lonnie, and Levine, Linda. *Shared Intimacies*. New York: Bantam Books, 1980.

Bing, Elizabeth, and Coleman, Libby. *Making Love During Pregnancy*. New York: Bantam Books, 1983.

Boston Women's Health Book Collective. *The New Our Bodies, Ourselves: A Book by and for Women*. New York: Simon & Schuster, 1984.

Burns, David. *Intimate Connections*. New York: Signet, 1985.

Butler, Robert and Lewis, Myrna. *Love and Sex After Sixty*. New York: Harper & Row, 1977.

———. *Love and Sex After Forty*. New York: Harper & Row, 1986.

Calderone, Mary, and Johnson, Eric. *The Family Book About Sexuality*. New York: Bantam Books, 1983.

Carrerra, Michael. *Sex: The Facts, the Acts, and Your Feelings*. New York: Crown, 1981.

Gordon, Sol, and Gordon, Judith. *Raising a Child Conservatively in a Sexually Permissive World*. New York: Simon & Schuster, 1983.

Levine, Linda, and Barbach, Lonnie. *The Intimate Male*. Garden City, N.Y.: Doubleday & Co., 1983.

Masters, William; Johnson, Virginia; and Kolodny, Robert. *Masters and Johnson on Sex and Human Loving*. Boston: Little, Brown & Co., 1986.

McCarthy, Barry, and McCarthy, Emily. *Sex and Satisfaction After Thirty*. Englewood Cliffs, N.J.: Prentice-Hall, 1981.

————. *Sexual Awareness: Sharing Sexual Pleasure*. New York: Carroll & Graf, 1984.

Schover, Leslie. *Prime Time: Sexual Health for Men Over Fifty*. Holt, Rinehart, and Winston, 1984.

Zilbegeld, Bernie. *Male Sexuality*. New York: Bantam Books, 1978.

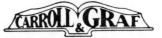

FINE WORKS OF NON-FICTION AVAILABLE IN QUALITY PAPERBACK EDITIONS FROM CARROLL & GRAF

- [ ] Anderson, Nancy/WORK WITH PASSION — $9.95
- [ ] Blanch, Lesley/THE WILDER SHORES OF LOVE — $8.95
- [ ] Cherry-Garrard/THE WORST JOURNEY IN THE WORLD — $13.95
- [ ] Conot, Robert/JUSTICE AT NUREMBURG — $11.95
- [ ] Cooper, Duff/OLD MEN FORGET — $10.95
- [ ] De Jonge, Alex/THE LIFE AND TIMES OF GRIGORII RASPUTIN — $10.95
- [ ] Elkington, John/THE GENE FACTORY — $8.95
- [ ] Garbus, Martin/TRAITORS AND HEROES — $10.95
- [ ] Golenbock, Peter/HOW TO WIN AT ROTISSERIE BASEBALL — $8.95
- [ ] Harris, A./SEXUAL EXERCISES FOR WOMEN — $8.95
- [ ] Hook, Sidney/OUT OF STEP — $14.95
- [ ] Keating, H. R. F./CRIME & MYSTERY: THE 100 BEST BOOKS — $7.95
- [ ] Lifton, David S./BEST EVIDENCE — $11.95
- [ ] Madden, David and Bach, Peggy/REDISCOVERIES II $9.95
- [ ] McCarthy, Barry and Emily/FEMALE SEXUAL AWARENESS — $9.95
- [ ] McCarthy, Barry & Emily/SEXUAL AWARENESS — $9.95
- [ ] Moorehead, Alan/THE RUSSIAN REVOLUTION — $10.95
- [ ] Morris, Charles/IRON DESTINIES, LOST OPPORTUNITIES: THE POST-WAR ARMS RACE — $13.95
- [ ] Stanway, Andrew/THE ART OF SENSUAL LOVING $15.95
- [ ] Trench, Charles/THE ROAD TO KHARTOUM — $10.95
- [ ] White, Jon Manchip/CORTES — $10.95
- [ ] Wilson, Colin/THE MAMMOTH BOOK OF TRUE CRIME — $8.95

Available from fine bookstores everywhere or use-this coupon for ordering.

Carroll & Graf Publishers, Inc., 260 Fifth Avenue, N.Y., N.Y. 10001
Please send me the books I have checked above. I am enclosing
$_____ (please add $1.00 per title to cover postage and
handling.) Send check or money order—no cash or C.O.D.'s
please. N.Y. residents please add 8¼% sales tax.

Mr/Mrs/Ms _____

Address _____

City _____ State/Zip _____
Please allow four to six weeks for delivery.